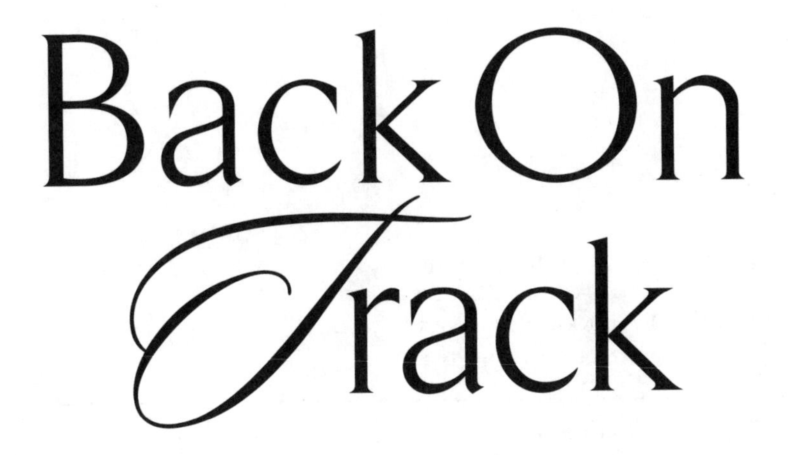

CAROLE LEWIS

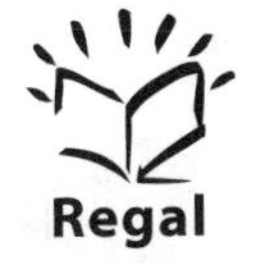

From Gospel Light
Ventura, California, U.S.A.

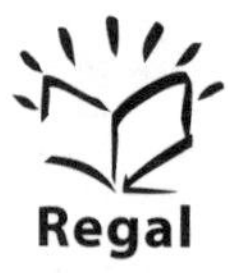

PUBLISHED BY REGAL BOOKS
FROM GOSPEL LIGHT
VENTURA, CALIFORNIA, U.S.A.
PRINTED IN THE U.S.A.

Regal Books is a ministry of Gospel Light, an evangelical Christian publisher dedicated to serving the local church. We believe God's vision for Gospel Light is to provide church leaders with biblical, user-friendly materials that will help them evangelize, disciple and minister to children, youth and families.

It is our prayer that this Regal book will help you discover biblical truth for your own life and help you meet the needs of others. May God richly bless you.

For a free catalog of resources from Regal Books/Gospel Light, please call your Christian supplier or contact us at 1-800-4-GOSPEL *or* www.regalbooks.com.

Cover and interior design by Robert Williams
Edited by Stephanie Jackson Parrish

ISBN 0-8307-3258-6

DEDICATION

I met Pat Lewis more than 30 years ago at church. She and her husband, Bill, and their three children had just moved to Houston from Arkansas. My earliest recollection of Pat and her family took place in church, as they sat in front of my family: I watched her daughter Tamara, then a toddler, wiggle in her ruffled-seat panties. As our friendship grew, I had the privilege of staying by Pat's side when her son Tim broke his neck at school. We rejoiced together as God mended Tim's neck. I grew to love Pat's oldest son, Terry, when I worked with him in the youth department of our church. In July 2000, when Bill went home to be with the Lord, Pat was already working in the First Place offices. I had begged her for years to come work with First Place, and the day she finally said yes was one of the highlights of my life. I have watched Pat grow and blossom in Christ during the years of our friendship. We have totally opposite personalities, and God has used this mightily in our working relationship. I push her, and she holds me back.

I am dedicating this book to Pat because God has used her more than any other person in my life to help me get back on track when I derail. She has been there for me through laughter and pain. She always encourages and never criticizes. She is the person behind the scenes, quietly working to make a woman like me look good.

She sweetly makes me plan, clean off my desk and pray before writing or calling someone when I'm angry or annoyed. Her wisdom and knowledge of the Scriptures is astounding. I have never known anyone who works harder or loves deeper than Pat Lewis.

Thank you, precious friend, for investing in my life.
I love you.
Carole

CONTENTS

Note to the Reader

Dear Reader,

I believe God has spoken to me truths about losing weight. I present these truths to you here, in *Back on Track.* Part 1 describes the battle we are in—the battle of the bulge—and brings the encouragement that God knows and cares where we've been, where we are and where we're going. Part 2 explains the Triple Dare, which is the 16-week plan that God gave me to lose weight—a simplified version of the First Place food plan. See chapter 8 for the fun origin of its name and its philosophical background. Appendix A details the plan.

I wanted to be open with you about my struggle with weight loss, so I wrote *Back on Track* while I was going through my own Triple Dare. For that reason, you'll see references such as "This week" and "I am in week 12 of my Triple Dare." I have also included, at the beginning of each chapter, the daily journal that I kept. As you read and respond to the message of this book, I hope you feel that you are journeying with me.

Also, you'll see many references to my mom, who was being cared for by hospice nurses while I was writing. My mom, Frances Juliet Harper, danced into heaven on January 3, 2003, at the age of 89.

Blessings,
Carole

INTRODUCTION

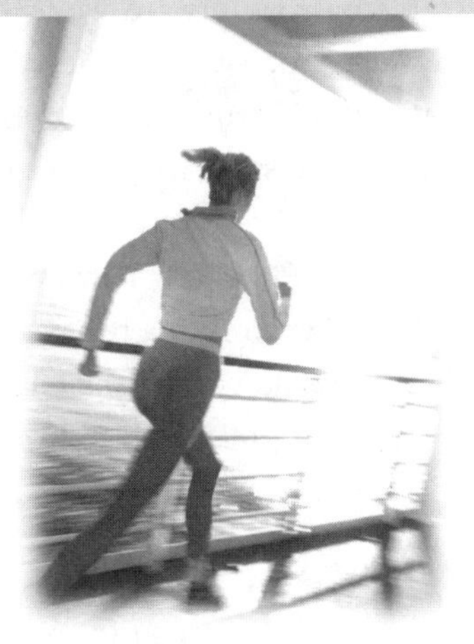

Those of us who are overweight have at least two things in common. The first is that we think about our weight most of the time. The second is that we wonder if today will be the day we decide to get back on track and start losing weight again. Many books have been written about weight loss, but most have been written by authorities in the field—people who know what we need to do and tell us how to do it.

A fellow struggler is writing this book. When it comes to losing weight and keeping it off, I identify most with the apostle Paul, who wrote in Romans 7:15-18:

> I do not understand what I do. For what I want to do I do not do, but what I hate I do. And if I do what I do not want to do, I agree that the law is good. As it is, it is no longer I myself who do it, but it is sin living in me. I know that nothing good lives in me, that is, in my sinful nature. For I have the desire to do what is good, but I cannot carry it out.

If you have purchased this book and need hope today that God cares about your plight, then you have picked up a book that quite possibly could change your life. I can say this with certainty, not because of any wisdom I possess, but because of the great power of God to change lives.

It is my prayer for each of us that from this day forward we will decide that God is big enough and powerful enough to be believed, trusted and obeyed. Together, as we accept these three truths and act on them, we will witness a miracle take place in our lives: We will discover the way to lose weight and to keep it off forever.

Even better than that, we will start experiencing God in a new way. As we learn how to believe, trust and obey, we will enter into a relationship with Him that is deeper than any we have ever had before—the relationship of a trusting child who has the most loving, gracious Daddy in the world.

PART ONE

THE BATTLE OF THE BULGE

Carole's Triple Dare Journal

Week 1

Starting weight: 160

Day 1 Monday, September 9, 2002

Dailiness: went to see Mom
Time spent: 1 hour
Accountability tip: measured peanut butter for my toast; found ½ tablespoon is perfect—only counts as ½ meat and ½ fat!

Day 2 Tuesday, September 10, 2002

Dailiness: forgot to set alarm; woke up late
Time lost: 2 hours
Accountability tip: measured to be sure I was eating ½ cup cereal

Day 3 Wednesday, September 11, 2002

Dailiness: cleaned toilet before I left for work (have thought about it for two days)
Time spent: 1 minute
Accountability tip: decided to share my plan next week at the national conference in Hattiesburg

Day 4 Thursday, September 12, 2002

Dailiness: great quiet time
Time spent: 1 hour
Time saved: unable to measure
Accountability tip: got a to-go box at lunch for half of 8″ veggie pizza; gave it to Lisa when I got back to work

Day 5 Friday, September 13, 2002

Dailiness: hospital, while friend Lynda had cancer surgery
Time spent: 4 hours
Accountability tip: meat at lunch, so ate a big salad with lots of veggies for dinner

Day 6 Saturday, September 14, 2002

Dailiness: boating; Johnny drove while I rode on the Triple Dare with my 20-year-old granddaughter, Cara, and her roommate, Katy—what fun!
Time spent: 4 hours
Accountability tip: ate out for lunch—four grilled shrimp with rice pilaf (ordered from appetizer menu)

Day 7 Sunday, September 15, 2002

Dailiness: went to church; signed *Today Is the First Day* between two worship services
Time spent: 5 hours
Accountability tip: had a big lunch, so had six crackers with 1 tablespoon peanut butter for dinner

CHAPTER 1

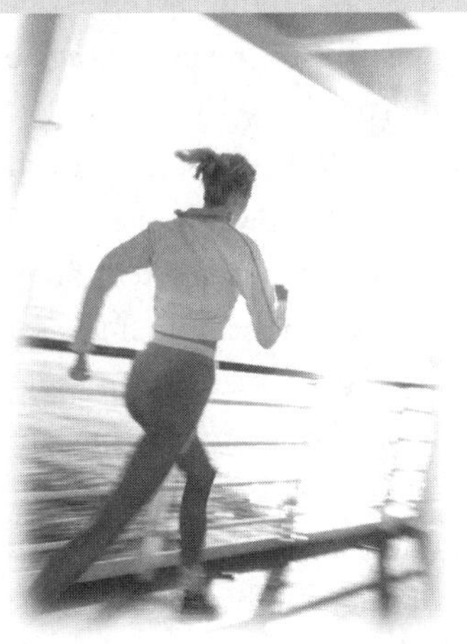

Dear friends, I urge you as aliens and strangers in the world, to abstain from sinful desires, which war against your soul.

1 PETER 2:11

This Is a War

Our Weapons Have Failed

The person who coined the phrase "the battle of the bulge" certainly knew what he or she was talking about. Until we understand that losing weight is a battle—that only God can fight and win—we will be doomed to failure. When we accept Jesus Christ as our Savior, our souls are secure and destined to live in heaven for eternity. Our bodies are quite another thing, just as Christ spoke of in Matthew 26:41: "The spirit is willing, but the body is weak." If we rely on our own power to bring our bodies into submission to God, we fail miserably. This is why trying to exercise *self-control* in weight loss has failed so many people, including myself. We can do it for a while, but never long enough to achieve permanent victory over this battle of the bulge.

Knowledge alone is not the answer either. Most of us own quite a few "war manuals" on weight loss, yet here we sit today staring defeat in the face. If spending *money* were the solution to this battle, most of us would have certainly won the war by now. The percentage of our own personal budgets that many of us have spent is comparable to the percentage of the federal government's budget spent on defense.

One of my dear friends, Beverly Henson, has lost 147 pounds in the First Place program and has kept it off for five years. Beverly is an entertaining speaker, and she keeps everyone in stitches when she tells about the thousands of dollars she spent trying to lose weight. When she saw Oprah Winfrey on television sharing that she had lost weight drinking a liquid six times a day, Beverly immediately signed up to do the same thing. She said she was doing really great until they started reintroducing solid food back into her diet. She calls it refeeding. When the refeeding started, she promptly gained back all the weight she had lost. Another time, Beverly was watching television and she saw a television evangelist with a healing ministry. She was a new Christian and, upon seeing this program, became convinced that she needed healing or she would never lose weight. So she chartered a 48-passenger bus, loaded it up with her friends and drove to the city where the preacher was holding a healing service. Beverly said her hopes were dashed when she was told that they were only taking people in wheelchairs that night!

All of us have stories about our weight-loss adventures and the money we have spent without finding the success we so desperately want. So, if *self-control*, *knowledge* and *money* will not help us win this battle of the bulge, where do we start? Let us look at some of the practical truths of any war.

We Wage War on More Than One Front

When we wage war against our weight without considering every aspect of our being, we are doomed to fail every time. So many of the diets we try wage war only on the physical. The weight appears to be the problem, so we attack it with another diet. But wars are waged on many different fronts—land, sea, air and covert operations. Likewise, if we focus only on "calories in, calories out," and yet fail to recognize the truth that we are four-sided—body, soul, mind and spirit—then we are waging war only on one front.

What areas (or fronts) will God (the master of covert operations) use to help us win the war?

1. Our bodies (the physical front)
2. Our minds (the mental front)
3. Our souls (the emotional front)
4. Our spirits (the spiritual front)

We Can Lose Battles and Still Win the War

In our weight-loss battle, we desire victory to be quick and easy; but wars are fought strategically—one battle at a time—and we must expect set-backs and defeats along the way.

Recently, I received a letter from a friend telling me about her weight-loss battle. She joined First Place weighing over 200 pounds. She had great success and soon found herself leading the group. Within eight months she had lost 80 pounds. Due to a series of circumstances, her First Place group stopped meeting for a while; she began a down-ward spiral and the weight began to creep back up again. Before long, she had gained back 40 pounds. This story has a happy ending because she is again in First Place and is losing the regained pounds.

If we are ever going to gain victory in the war of our bodies against our spirits, we must understand that we will lose battles along the way. I want more than anything to be a woman of God; but if I refuse to believe that I am fighting a spiritual battle, then I will be one of the first casualties and will be disqualified for the victory celebration. Paul said it this way in 1 Corinthians 9:27: "I beat my body and make it my slave so that after I have preached to others, I myself will not be disqualified for the prize." If we can learn how to give God permission to fight this bat-tle that we are waging, we will find the keys to victory.

On September 9, 2002, God called me to the battle to lose the weight that I needed to lose. He asked me to do this as I write this book so that

I can share the truths that He is teaching me on the way to victory. I had six wonderful weeks and found that I had lost weight when I got on the scale each Monday.

In week seven, I flew to California with my husband, Johnny, for a doctor's appointment. Just like Paul Prudhomme (the wonderful, well-known New Orleans chef whose recipes Johnny loves) creates recipes that are complicated and must be followed to the letter, so Johnny's doctor gives instructions that are complicated and must be followed to the letter for Johnny's treatment to be effective. My mind must stay alert

We will lose some battles,
but if we allow God to have control,
He will help us win the war.

when I take notes for the minimum of five hours that we are at the doctor's office each time. So, after six hours in the doctor's office this time, we were both tired and hungry.

As we left the doctor's office at 7:30 P.M., Johnny remembered a sushi restaurant close by in Santa Monica. We went inside and Johnny ordered sushi. Being tired, I let my defenses down and ordered shrimp and vegetable tempura. I did not even look closely at the menu to see what other options I might choose. Tempura would not have been such a bad choice, but God and I had launched this war with two absolute directives: Do not eat any fried food, and do not eat any high-calorie, high-sugar, high-fat desserts. (I want the plan in this book to be simple, though not easy.) After eating the tempura, I could have gotten right back on track the next morning. I didn't though; I ordered tempura once more while we were in Ventura. When I got on the scale Monday to begin week eight, I had gained one pound. Here was my opportunity to quit or to decide to get back on track that very minute. I am happy to say that

I was able to get back on track. Week eight was a new week, a fresh start. It would be different from week seven because I had learned a valuable truth that I had heard quoted: If we don't learn from history, we are destined to repeat it.

Johnny told me that he once heard a weight "expert" on a popular talk show say, "The battle to lose weight is not a sprint, it's a marathon." Everyone clapped and loved this statement. Even the host said, "That's good!" As Johnny sat there and thought about that statement, he said to himself, *A marathon ends after 26.2 miles, but the battle to lose weight never ends.* As he relayed the statement to me, he said, "Ask an alcoholic or a drug addict if their battle is a marathon. They will tell you that their battle doesn't have an end." After thinking about what Johnny said, I realized that, yes, this is an ongoing battle—with very real victories and very real defeats. We will want to remember that we will lose some battles, but if we allow God to have control, He will help us win the war.

We Must Recognize Our Weaknesses

I joined the First Place program in March of 1981 and have led First Place groups since I finished that first session. As the director of the program, I have been privileged to meet hundreds of men and women who have joined the fight. Some have lost over 200 pounds and have been able to keep it off for years. They all say that there are still skirmishes, even though they have obtained victory in losing weight. They also say that, at any point, they could easily let their defenses down and start gaining weight again.

It is my belief that the reason for this is that people who have lost and gained weight for years are compulsive overeaters. Those of us who are compulsive overeaters know it. Once we get started eating a high-calorie food, we feel we must finish the entire container before we can get back on track. We may eat it all at one sitting or eat it every day until we decide just to finish it and get it out of the house. Throwing the food in the trash is usually not an option we choose. For some, the food is crunchy and salty. Others, like me, are drawn to creamy and sweet foods.

Compulsive overeating doesn't hinge on whether we have a little or a lot of weight to lose. When we overeat compulsively, getting back on track is harder. It keeps us from having victory over the food we eat. Our emotions get into the mix, and we again lose hope that we can ever change permanently. God wants to help us overcome this destructive habit, so it is imperative that we recognize ourselves as compulsive overeaters and ask Him for help.

A lady in this session of my First Place class weighed in at over 200 pounds the first week. She has a stressful job (who doesn't?), and she told me at the end of the first week that she had written God a letter. In the letter she said, "O God, you do have a sense of humor. In the past I overate when I was stressed; now I can't even do that!" I never heard a truer statement. The best part of this story is that she recognizes why she overeats. Until we recognize that we have a problem, we will never ask for help.

I can count on one hand the people I have known over the years who joined First Place because they needed to learn how to eat right. One of these women came into the program, and I asked her at the first meeting when her baby was due. Since she was wearing a maternity top, I *assumed* (which is, by the way, the lowest form of knowledge) that she was pregnant. She said, "My baby is six months old and that's why I'm here." She lost the excess weight she had gained while pregnant and never came back to First Place. Since she is a member of my church and I see her from time to time, I am always struck by the fact that for the last 18 years she has not gained back the weight she lost in that one session of First Place.

If you are like this woman, you probably are not interested in reading this book. The book isn't being written for those who need knowledge. There is enough knowledge out there today for us to lose all the weight we need to lose. If you are reading this book and you realize that this battle of the bulge is an ongoing battle that will be hard to win—but not impossible—then you have overcome the biggest hurdle of the war.

Let's Not Give Up

To win this battle of the bulge we must remain confident, strong and relentless. The difference in this war, though, is that our confidence will need to be placed in God and not in ourselves, where it has been in the past. We must be confident that God's Word, the Bible, is true and that we can believe it. We must be strong as we make the conscious choice to believe that God is able to fight this battle and to trust Him for the victory—even after apparent defeat on some days. Being relentless means that we will say with Winston Churchill, in his famous speech of 1941 at Harrow School, "Never give in. Never give in. Never, never, never, never—in nothing great or small, large or petty—never give in, except to convictions of honour and good sense. Never yield to force. Never yield to the apparently overwhelming might of the enemy."[1]

Our confidence will need to be placed in God and not in ourselves, where it has been in the past.

At the end of the Gulf War, we—as well as the news reporters—were amazed to hear that the Iraqi fighters were giving up to anyone they met along the way. The reason for their surrender is summed up in these seven words: *They had lost the will to fight.* You may be reading these words right now and thinking, *That's me. I have fought a good fight, but I have lost so many battles that I am ready to give up.* The very fact that you are reading this book is evidence that you still want to fight. Our enemy, the devil, wants us to believe that we will never win; but God's Word says, "I press on toward the goal to *win* the prize for which God has called me heavenward in Christ Jesus" (Phil. 3:14, emphasis added). Ultimate victory will be achieved on the day we go home to heaven. In order to have victory on a daily basis we must believe that God wants us to have victory in the here and now. To secure victory on this earth, we must learn the secrets that all good soldiers know instinctively and remember that God will never be able to help us win our own personal battles if we refuse to fight.

As we move on to chapter 2, let us remember these truths:

1. Wars are fought strategically, one battle at a time.
2. Wars are fought on more than one front.
3. Recognizing our own weaknesses will help us win the war.
4. We must expect setbacks and defeats along the way.
5. When we lose a battle, we must get back on track immediately, so we don't lose the war.
6. We will not win if we refuse to fight.

Put on your uniform. We are now ready to start basic training!

PRAYER

Dear Lord, I admit that this weight I need to lose is a problem I cannot handle myself. Come into my life today in might and power. Give me the strength to get up and fight this war, knowing that You will help me fight. Help me believe that as You give me the strength to fight, I will win, if I do not quit. In Jesus' name, amen.

WEEK 2

Weight: 157½ **Loss:** 2½ pounds

DAY 8 MONDAY, SEPTEMBER 16, 2002

Dailiness: stayed late (First Place council meeting)
Time spent: 5 hours
Accountability tip: I am soooooo sore from Saturday's ride on Triple Dare! Maybe 60-year-old women should rethink doing this!!!

DAY 9 TUESDAY, SEPTEMBER 17, 2002

Dailiness: spoke at First Place luncheon
Time spent: 2 hours
Accountability tip: didn't try everything at luncheon; only ate what I could count

DAY 10 WEDNESDAY, SEPTEMBER 18, 2002

Dailiness: got ready for national conference
Time spent: 10 hours
Accountability tip: ate big salad for lunch; resisted carrot salad on salad bar

DAY 11 THURSDAY, SEPTEMBER 19, 2002

Dailiness: packed to go to Hattiesburg—national First Place conference
Time spent: 2 hours
Accountability tip: split dinner with Kay

DAY 12 FRIDAY, SEPTEMBER 20, 2002

Dailiness: walked with friends at conference
Time spent: 45 minutes
Accountability tip: ordered baked potato and salad for lunch

DAY 13 SATURDAY, SEPTEMBER 21, 2002

Dailiness: packed, drove to airport, flew home—left cell phone in rental car!
Time spent: 4 hours
Accountability tip: threw away cookie in box lunch at conference

DAY 14 SUNDAY, SEPTEMBER 22, 2002

Dailiness: got up at 3 A.M. to write
Time spent: 4 hours
Accountability tip: had strawberry-and-orange-juice smoothie for breakfast

CHAPTER 2

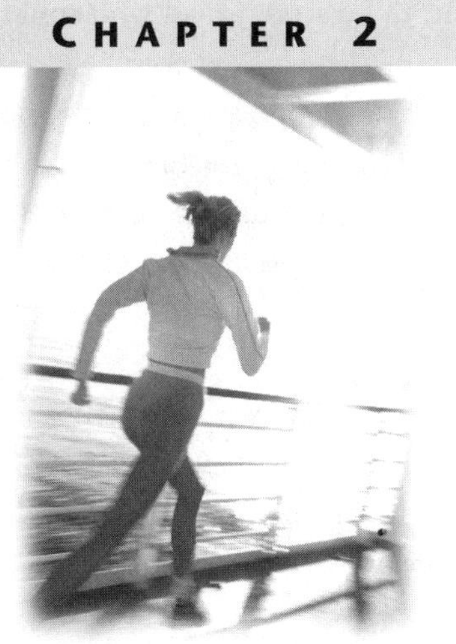

You know my folly, O God;
my guilt is not hidden from you.

PSALM 69:5

GOD KNOWS WHERE WE'VE BEEN

When our son, John, was about four years old, he and a little neighbor boy ventured across a busy street to play in a dirt pile. When we realized that John was missing, my husband, Johnny, and I started to look for him. Before we found them, John and his friend came walking back into our yard; they were covered with dirt. I will never forget the conversation between daddy and son that day. My husband, knowing that there was a pile of dirt on the other side of the busy street, said to John, "Did you two boys go across Voss Road?" The boys looked sheepish and shook their heads no. Johnny then said, "That looks like Voss Road dirt to me. Are you sure you didn't cross Voss Road?" At this point both boys confessed that they had been across the road playing in the pile of dirt. I will never forget the amazed look on John's face when my husband seemed to recognize the dirt. My son's expression conveyed that he thought his dad must have been the smartest man in the world—a man who could tell where dirt comes from!

I have thought about that scene many times over the years. To me the story illustrates the very real fact that *God knows where we've been.* God knows, not just because He can see the dirt all over us, but because He saw the dirt pile in the first place. God knows because He is God. Psalm 139:15-16 says,

> My frame was not hidden from you when I was made in the secret place. When I was woven together in the depths of the earth, your eyes saw my unformed body. All the days ordained for me were written in your book before one of them came to be.

God knows where we've been. He knows all the crazy things we've tried because we wanted to lose weight. He knows that as we have struggled on our own to lose weight, our minds, emotions and bodies have gotten dirty.

God knows all the crazy things we've tried because we wanted to lose weight.

Our minds have been sullied because we've believed that to be of any worth in this world, we must be thin. The society we live in tells us, without saying it in so many words, that only the thin are clean; the fat are unclean. Magazines portray thin movie stars with shining hair and radiant skin, while the overweight movie stars look like they need a good bath. Tabloids love to make a cover story of catching an overweight star looking sweaty and sloppily dressed. Because our minds are constantly bombarded with these images of thin people as beautiful and fat people as ugly, we have bought into this lie.

Our emotions have been soiled because we continue to fail. We've spent money that our family needed for other things—not once, but many times—so that we could try some new diet that we fail, just like the other ones. In fact, we even *feel* dirty. When we allow our feelings to take control, they tell us that because of our past history of failure, we will never succeed at losing weight, so we may as well just give in and give up. Our feelings keep us in a helpless, hopeless state. We desperately want success, but we feel like failures.

Our bodies are dingy because we've done so many crazy things to lose weight that some of us have a metabolism that no longer works properly. We are coping with diseases like diabetes or heart disease, many times brought on by the foods we have eaten and our lack of physical exercise.

God knows everywhere that we have been and everything that we have done up to this point. My prayer for you and for me is that we tell God right now that we're aware that He knows how dirty we feel and then ask Him to clean the dirt of unbelief from our minds, bodies and spirits. That's when He will be able to bring about the needed changes we so desire.

Prayer

Dear Father, You know all the foolish things I have done to lose weight. Help me today to believe that You want to help me lose all the weight necessary to be healthy so that I am able to serve You with my whole heart. Help me to trust You to show me how, and then help me to obey You completely. In Jesus' name, amen.

WEEK 3

Weight: 155 **Loss:** 2½ pounds

DAY 15 MONDAY, SEPTEMBER 23, 2002

Dailiness: stayed home to pack for Hurricane Isador
Time spent: all day
Accountability tip: ate out; ordered from sides menu

DAY 16 TUESDAY, SEPTEMBER 24, 2002

Dailiness: planted fall flowers
Time spent: 5 hours
Accountability tip: gave half of turkey poor-boy sandwich to Johnny

DAY 17 WEDNESDAY, SEPTEMBER 25, 2002

Dailiness: haircut
Time spent: 1 hour
Accountability tip: split entrée with Pat at lunch

DAY 18 THURSDAY, SEPTEMBER 26, 2002

Dailiness: cleaned for Saturday's Sunday School party at my house
Time spent: all day
Accountability tip: split dinner with Johnny

DAY 19 FRIDAY, SEPTEMBER 27, 2002

Dailiness: washed windows
Time spent: 4 hours
Accountability tip: split lunch with Pat

DAY 20 SATURDAY, SEPTEMBER 28, 2002

Dailiness: party at our house
Time spent: 8 A.M.-8 P.M.
Accountability tip: ate fresh fruit instead of desserts

DAY 21 SUNDAY, SEPTEMBER 29, 2002

Dailiness: stayed at church all day to get e-mails caught up (out most of last week)
Time spent: 4 hours
Accountability tip: had big lunch, light supper

CHAPTER 3

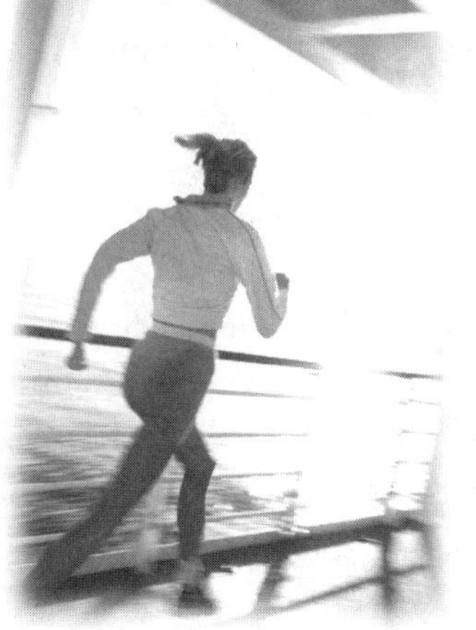

If I say, "Surely the darkness will hide me and the light become night around me," even the darkness will not be dark to you; the night will shine like the day, for darkness is as light to you.

PSALM 139:11-12

GOD KNOWS WHERE WE ARE

One Saturday morning after shopping at my local grocery store, I placed my groceries in the trunk, got in the car and sat there for a few minutes looking at my grocery receipt and thinking that I had been overcharged for a particular sale item. When I finally put the receipt in my purse and started the car for the drive home, I was shocked to see that a dense fog had rolled in. All the way home I had my windshield wipers on, hoping to see far enough ahead to get home safely. Anyone who knows me knows that I usually drive too fast. That particular day, though, I was unable to drive faster than 10 miles per hour the entire three miles to my house. As I inched along, I watched the ditch on my right and the yellow stripe on my left to stay on my side of the road. When I finally got to the house, I breathed a sigh of relief and turned off the engine. Imagine my surprise when I opened the door of the car and saw nothing but blue sky and beautiful sunshine—except on the inside of my car!

I could not figure out what had happened until I remembered sitting in the car looking at that receipt. It all suddenly made sense; my breath had fogged the inside of the windows. I felt embarrassed when I thought about the number of people who might have seen me struggling to drive home in the dense fog of my own creation.

It has been said that our perception of reality is our reality. If we think we are in a fog, we are in a fog. I'm glad that my God is never in a fog. Even when the darkness of my present circumstances prevents me from seeing clearly, my darkness is not dark to God. God knows where we are this very minute. He knows where we're sitting, what we're thinking and what we might be eating; and He knows how we feel. Jesus said in Luke 12:7, "Indeed, the very hairs of your head are all numbered." Yes, God knows where we are.

Aren't you glad that God's view is different from the world's view? Our society is obsessed with top 10 lists. There are lists of the top 10 songs, the top 10 books, the 10 best dressed, the 10 best restaurants and so on. God is not the God of the top 10. He not only knows where I am, but He also has put every problem that I have as number 1 on His list. Whether it is a real problem or an imagined one, if it is a problem to me, God knows about it and has a solution. I find great comfort in this truth!

Likewise, God does not have a top 10 list of our mistakes, beginning with number 10, our smallest failure, and leading up to number 1, our greatest. Wherever we are today, God knows. He knows if we are miserable and overweight. He knows if we have a rotten marriage. He knows if our children are disobedient and out of control. He knows our problems and He knows our failures.

The most exciting part about God's knowing where we are right here, right now, is that He never condemns us or berates us for our failures or for our feelings of failure. If we are overweight, depressed and without hope today, God has good news for us. God knows all about your situation and mine, and those situations are not dark to Him. If we're feeling condemned instead of comforted by the knowledge that

God knows, then our belief system about God is faulty.

Instead of asking God to fix our problems and turn our failures into successes, most of us spend too much time blaming ourselves or somebody else for every situation in life. Having a little something to eat always makes us feel better–temporarily. As we gain more and more weight, the fog rolls in and we find ourselves enveloped in the darkness of our own choices. We find ourselves agreeing with the apostle Paul, who said in Romans 7:24, "What a wretched man I am! Who will rescue me from this body of death?"

As we gain more and more weight, the fog rolls in and we find ourselves enveloped in the darkness of our own choices.

We can be thankful today that God knows about our problems and our failures and that He worked out a plan to set us free. God sent His only Son, Jesus, to live in our world, to experience the same kind of pain we experience and to be tempted in all ways, just as we are tempted. The good news is that even though we fail the tests of life on a daily basis, Jesus did not fail. Jesus passed every test with flying colors. Because He was willing to die on a cross for our problems and failures, we have the opportunity to accept His sacrifice as the payment for every wrong thing we have ever done. When we do this and ask Jesus to come into our lives and take over, He immediately comes in to give us the power to overcome. The Holy Spirit of God comes to live in our hearts to teach us what to do and say and, yes, even what to eat.

If you have never asked Jesus to come into your heart and forgive you of your sin, you can pray this prayer right now and settle the most important issue of your life. This prayer is the starting point for believing, trusting and obeying God.

PRAYER

Dear God, I know that I have made many mistakes in my life, and I am sorry for every one. I ask You to forgive my sin and to come into my heart right now. I believe that Jesus died on the cross for my sin. I believe that Jesus was buried and rose again from the grave after three days. I believe that Jesus is in heaven today, sitting at Your right hand. I ask You to give me a new heart and help me become the person You want me to be. Thank you, God, for saving me. In Jesus' name, amen.

You may be reading these words and thinking, *I've already done that, so why am I in such a mess?* It goes right back to our belief system. We were able to muster up enough belief that God had the power to save us from our sin, but we still can't seem to believe that He wants to save us from our present perception of reality. Zig Ziglar said it best in his book *See You at the Top*: "You are the sum total of what goes into your mind"[1] In essence, you become what you usually think about.

We do not have to stay where we are today. God knows where we've been and He knows where we are. Why not thank God right now that He knows where you are and ask Him to fix your problems and failures for His glory.

PRAYER

Dear Father, I want to thank You that You know where I am today. Help me to believe, trust and obey You so that I can experience the needed changes in my life. In Jesus' name, amen.

WEEK 4

Weight: 153 3/4 **Loss:** 1 1/4 pounds

DAY 22 MONDAY, SEPTEMBER 30, 2002

Dailiness: worked out 6 A.M.
Time spent: 50 minutes
Accountability tip: Luby's lunch—corn casserole was my bread choice

DAY 23 TUESDAY, OCTOBER 1, 2002

Dailiness: led First Place class; stayed after work for evening Bible study
Time spent: 5 hours
Accountability tip: chef's salad for dinner, dressing on side

DAY 24 WEDNESDAY, OCTOBER 2, 2002

Dailiness: took Mom to doctor
Time spent: 3 hours
Accountability tip: baked potato and salad for dinner

DAY 25 THURSDAY, OCTOBER 3, 2002

Dailiness: new publicity pictures
Time spent: 3 hours
Accountability tip: business lunch—tortilla soup

DAY 26 FRIDAY, OCTOBER 4, 2002

Dailiness: errands
Time spent: 2 hours
Accountability tip: shared a dinner with Johnny

DAY 27 SATURDAY, OCTOBER 5, 2002

Dailiness: cleaned boat
Time spent: 4 hours
Accountability tip: had all my fat at lunch; ate pasta for supper

DAY 28 SUNDAY, OCTOBER 6, 2002

Dailiness: ran errands for Fitness Week in the afternoon
Time spent: 6 hours
Accountability tip: big lunch; soup for supper

CHAPTER 4

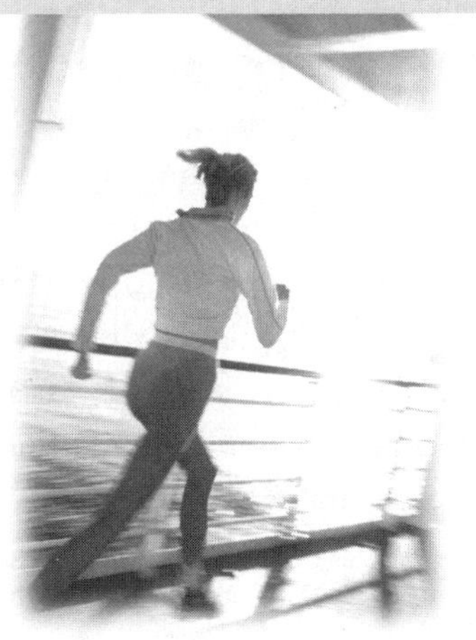

"For I know the plans I have for you," declares the LORD, "plans to prosper you and not to harm you, plans to give you hope and a future."

JEREMIAH 29:11

GOD KNOWS WHERE WE'RE GOING

My associate, Kay Smith, and I have traveled many miles together. Planning our trips has never been all that difficult. Kay corresponds with our host about the dates and times that we will be speaking. We purchase our airline tickets, pack our bags, board the airplane and usually arrive at our city of destination on time. The problem always seems to arise when we're sitting inside the rental car trying to decide which way to go in order to arrive at our final destination. We have been hopelessly lost so many times, only to find ourselves miraculously sitting in front of the church on time. One of our coworkers, Brenda, remarked, "I just know that every time you two get ready to leave town, the two angels God assigns to protect you beg God to send someone else!"

We're glad God knows where we're going, even when we don't. I have never seen it fail that when one of us has had a miserable past or a miserable present, God does His finest work. When we make the conscious decision to ask God to step into our mess and help us, a true miracle takes place: God uses our unpleasant past and present circumstances as a basis for our future ministry.

I know so many men and women who testify to the truth of this statement. Some women have had an abortion and God uses them as spokespersons for the pro-life movement. Some have suffered sexual abuse and God uses them to help other hurting men and women find healing. Recovered alcoholics or drug addicts are able to pull others

When we make the conscious decision to ask God to step into our mess and help us, a true miracle takes place: God uses our unpleasant past and present circumstances as a basis for our future ministry.

from that same pit. It is the same when we have struggled with being overweight for years. God knows where we've been, He knows where we are, and He knows where we're going. We can find hope if we will let these words sink into our minds. Many men and women who have struggled to lose weight for years have lost the weight and are victoriously leading First Place classes today. God is using the messes of their past as the basis for their ministry today.

Because God knows where we're going, it stands to reason that He would want us to go now rather than later. So what is stopping us? I know you're tired of hearing this, but the culprit lies in our belief system. It is much easier to believe that God knows where well-known Christian authors and Bible teachers—such as Beth Moore, Bruce Wilkinson, Kay Arthur or Chuck Swindoll—are going than to believe that He knows where we are going and that it's a better place than where we are right now. Our belief system is faulty when we believe that God has good plans for others but not for us. God doesn't love one person to a greater degree than He loves another. When God says in Jeremiah 29:11 that His plans are to prosper us and not harm us, He means just that.

One truth I have learned about God is that time is no big deal to Him. God has all the time in the world. Another truth I have learned is that He wants me to value the time given to me because I only have a certain number of years to live on this earth. I have seen God work mighty miracles in the lives of men and women in just a short year or two. In fact, look what God did through Jesus in the three short years of His earthly ministry. When we refuse to ask God to help us get back on track, we are basically implying that we enjoy living the way we are and we're not interested in permanent change.

Often we are so bound up in our present that we fail to stop and realize that God has wonderful things planned for our future. The dailiness of our lives keeps us from looking up or looking forward. We are so earthbound that we are sometimes no heavenly good. It is imperative that we understand that life is daily for everyone. Rich or poor, there are some things we all have in common. We all must tend to personal hygiene. On some mornings I look in the mirror and wish that I didn't have to wash my hair. When I have those thoughts, I immediately walk to the shower, turn on the water and get in. Once my hair is wet, I am committed to finishing the job. It's the same with most everything we do on a daily basis. Sometimes we spend more time fretting about our daily tasks than just doing them. God knows how daily our lives are and how earthbound we have become. He knows that if the enemy can keep us engrossed with the present challenges of each day, then we will never venture to peer into the wonderful future God has planned for us. We must not let the enemy capture us in this lie!

When my children were small, the daily grind was sometimes overwhelming. It seemed that my house was never clean. Toys were everywhere and there was always a mountain of clothes to wash. A wise Sunday School teacher helped me transport myself from my present situation and look toward the future when she said these words: "Your children will never remember when they are grown whether the house was clean all the time. They won't even remember what they had for dinner and how hard you worked to prepare it. They will remember the times you spent reading to them or praying with them." Those words turned me around and propelled me out of the present and right into my children's future. I no longer felt guilty if I sat and read to my children when there was housework to be done. I was investing in my children's future.

If we are to believe that God knows where we are going, then we must learn the difference between eternal significance and daily significance. Asking God to give me the opportunity to do something each day that will have eternal value makes my daily chores become less mundane. The enemy loves to keep us focused on the moment. When we worry and fret over all we have to do rather than give our dailiness to God and allow Him to arrange our day, we are destined to fail. God knows where we're going, and He wants to propel us into the future He has planned for us. Our job is to allow Him to work. Without our cooperation, this will never happen. Our daily grind is a great blessing from God. Without the dailiness of life, we would have little purpose. The problem comes when we focus so much on the present and lose sight of the future. Giving God my dailiness assures that my future will be what He has planned.

Prayer

Dear Father, I am comforted that You know where I'm going, even when I can't picture a bright future for myself. Help me to believe that Your plans for me are good and to trust You to bring them to pass in my life. In Jesus' name, amen.

Carole's Triple Dare Journal

Week 5

Weight: 152¾ **Loss:** 1 pound

Day 29 Monday, October 7, 2002

Dailiness: Mom in hospital
Time spent: 24 hours
Accountability tip: yogurt and fruit from grocery store

Day 30 Tuesday, October 8, 2002

Dailiness: hospital with Mom
Time spent: 5 hours
Accountability tip: grilled shrimp tacos; took two tortillas off

Day 31 Wednesday, October 9, 2002

Dailiness: hospital with Mom; drove to Round Top
Time spent: all day
Accountability tip: grilled chicken salad—no chips and salsa

Day 32 Thursday, October 10, 2002

Dailiness: Fitness Week begins
Time spent: all day
Accountability tip: ate only half of huge hamburger; left German potatoes

Day 33 Friday, October 11, 2002

Dailiness: Fitness Week
Time spent: all day
Accountability tip: no chips at lunch

Day 34 Saturday, October 12, 2002

Dailiness: Fitness Week
Time spent: all day
Accountability tip: no tastes or treats at Scarecrow Festival

Day 35 Sunday, October 13, 2002

Dailiness: Fitness Week
Time spent: all day
Accountability tip: ate 1,400 calories; no treats at Round Top

CHAPTER 5

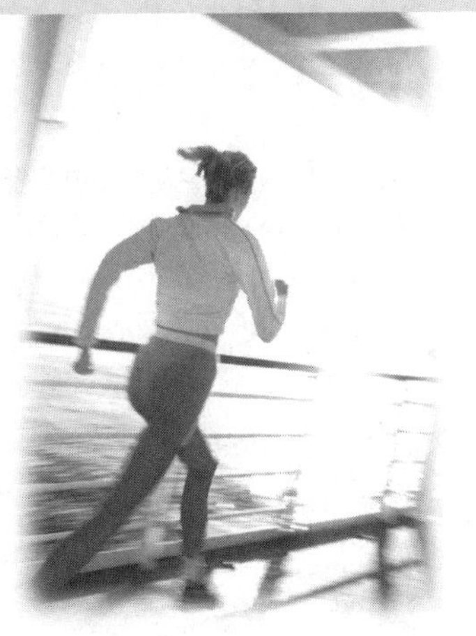

"Though the mountains be shaken and the hills be removed, yet my unfailing love for you will not be shaken nor my covenant of peace be removed," says the LORD, *who has compassion on you.*

ISAIAH 54:10

God Cares Where We've Been

Earthquakes in Our Past

In October and November 2002, the news media reported several occurrences of earthquakes. The most disturbing one was in Italy, where an entire class of first graders died. We sometimes experience things in life that make us feel as though we are being shattered; however, most of our earthquakes are small in comparison to the loss of life experienced by the families of those children. Nevertheless, our earthquakes are *our* earthquakes, and they shake us to the core when we're in the middle of them.

Perhaps you have experienced some horrendous earthquakes in your childhood, and life since that time has been one aftershock after another.

Struggles with our weight are part of the aftershock effect. I have good news for all of us today: God cares where we've been. He was there when we were going through the quake, and He hated every minute we suffered.

Others who struggle with being overweight may not have had any obvious abuse from childhood. Maybe their parents worked outside the home and they were latchkey children. Food was used for comfort when they felt lonely or afraid, and food is still being used today to bring comfort.

Still others had a wonderful childhood with loving parents who were overweight themselves. Food was always available and most times the food wasn't healthy. Habits were learned long ago that are hard to break.

We may never know the real reason we struggle with weight issues. The important thing is that God knows the reason and has the power to help us overcome any struggles that we've faced in the past, that we face today or that we may face in the future. As we learn how to give Christ first place in our lives, He will give us victory where we once knew only defeat.

Oswald Chambers said, "If you are going to be used by God, He will take you through a number of experiences that are not meant for you personally at all. They are designed to make you useful in His hands, and to enable you to understand what takes place in the lives of others."[1]

God wants to use the earthquakes of our past, along with the aftershocks of our present, to get us where He intends for us to be. To find that place, we must learn to say with the apostle Peter, "But rejoice that you participate in the sufferings of Christ, so that you may be overjoyed when his glory is revealed" (1 Pet. 4:13).

Recently, I wrote a letter to the men and women who took the 16-week Triple Dare along with me. I shared how I gained a pound one week from eating tempura not once but twice while in California. Here is one of the e-mails I received in response:

> I, too, gained one-half pound this week. I went to a luncheon and shouldn't have eaten what was served, but I did and it was a very high-fat meal. Instead of getting right back on track immediately,

> I went to my children's ball game that night and drank two large hot chocolates. That was very smart! Nevertheless, I am back on track 100 percent.

I have received several more e-mails that relate the same type of incident. I believe God is trying to tell us something here. He not only cares where we've been, but He also cares when we go back there again.

PRISONERS OF THE PAST

In chapter 1, I said that losing weight and keeping it off is a war. I didn't write that it *was* a war, but that it *is* a war. When we go back to the quake scene, we get off track; many of us stay off track for months or years before we make the conscious decision to leave the quake area forever. The apostle Paul said in Galatians 5:1, "It is for freedom that Christ has set us free. Stand firm, then, and do not let yourselves be burdened again by a yoke of slavery." Yes, you and I will go back to the quake site from time to time, but we don't have to stay there.

Recently, on my drive into work, I heard a wonderful message by Captain Charlie Plum on Focus on the Family's radio broadcast. Captain Plum told about his plane getting shot down over Vietnam just five days before his eight-month tour of duty was over. He spent six horrendous years in prison camps before being rescued. Charlie had a breakthrough when another high-level American prisoner reached out to him. The two of them talked back and forth in their adjacent cells by using a code. Because Charlie weighed 115 pounds and had boils all over his body, he was not upbeat about what he had endured. Charlie shared with his new friend that everything happening was not his fault and did not seem fair. His friend told him something profound: "Charlie, you are suffering from a disease that has killed many prisoners, and that disease is called prison thinking."[2]

Becoming "burdened again by a yoke of slavery" (Gal. 5:1) means that we are consciously putting ourselves back into the concentration camp of our past. Even though the war of our past is over, we continue to think like a prisoner. Since concentration camps do not have an abundance of food, we always make sure that food is in abundance when we travel back to our experience. After we have started eating out of control, whether it is two tempura meals or two large hot chocolates, we always have the opportunity to make a conscious choice. We can continue on

God will set us free from the prison of our past so that we can remain free forever.

this destructive path we have chosen, or we can choose to believe that God cares where we've been and that He will set us free from our prison so that we can remain free forever. We must choose to get back on track every time we want to go back to that prison of our past or to the frustration of our present.

Do we really believe that God cares about where we've been? If so, let us tell God today that we're sick and tired of being a prisoner of our past. Let us choose to believe that God cares where we have been and tell Him right now that we want to be free from the aftershocks of our past once and for all.

Prayer

Dear Father, thank You that You were in my past. You hurt for me and You cared. Thank You that You still care today about where I've been and that You have the power to help me move forward from where I am today. Help me to believe that You care for me and help me to trust You for help to make the needed changes in my life. In Jesus' name, amen.

WEEK 6
Weight: 151½ **Loss:** 1¼ pounds

DAY 36 MONDAY, OCTOBER 14, 2002
Dailiness: Fitness Week
Time spent: all day
Accountability tip: no cheese or sour cream on fajitas

DAY 37 TUESDAY, OCTOBER 15, 2002
Dailiness: Fitness Week
Time spent: all day
Accountability tip: asked for forgiveness for sharp tongue

DAY 38 WEDNESDAY, OCTOBER 16, 2002
Dailiness: Fitness Week
Time spent: all day
Accountability tip: spoke on personal accountability

DAY 39 THURSDAY, OCTOBER 17, 2002
Dailiness: Fitness Week
Time spent: all day
Accountability tip: 37 people together lost 115 pounds

DAY 40 FRIDAY, OCTOBER 18, 2002
Dailiness: chauffeured Patsy Clairmont
Time spent: all day
Accountability tip: ate peanut butter sandwich at office

DAY 41 SATURDAY, OCTOBER 19, 2002
Dailiness: hospital with Mom
Time spent: 5 hours
Accountability tip: no snacks from vending machine

DAY 42 SUNDAY, OCTOBER 20, 2002
Dailiness: hospital with Mom
Time spent: 6 hours
Accountability tip: snack—dry box of raisin bran with coffee at hospital

CHAPTER 6

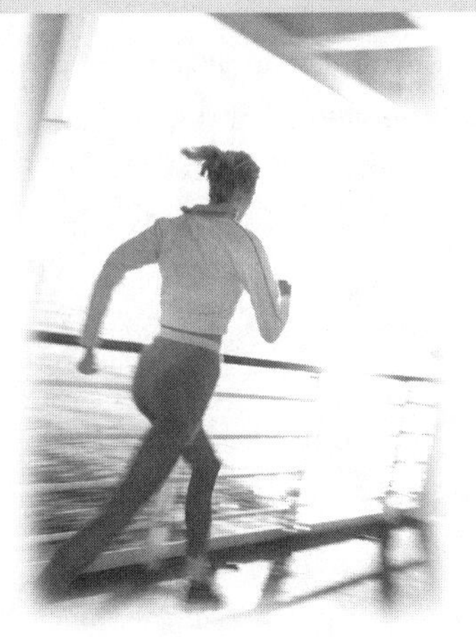

Cast all your anxiety on him because he cares for you.

1 PETER 5:7

GOD CARES WHERE WE ARE

Let's take a quiz:

1. Name the five wealthiest people in the world.
2. Name the last five Heisman Trophy winners.
3. Name the last five winners of the Miss America contest.
4. Name the last five winners of the Nobel Prize.

The point is, few of us remember the headliners of yesterday. If you knew the names of the people above, they were no second-rate achievers. They were the best in their fields. The truth is that applause dies, awards tarnish and achievements are forgotten.

Here's another quiz. Let's see how we do on this one:

1. List a few teachers who aided your journey through school.
2. Name three friends who have each helped you through a difficult time.
3. Name five people who have taught you something worthwhile.
4. Think of a few people who have made you feel appreciated and special.
5. Think of five people you enjoy spending time with.
6. Name half a dozen heroes whose stories have inspired you.

Wasn't that easier? What's the lesson?

The people who make a difference in life are not the ones with the most credentials, the most money or the most awards. The people who make a difference in life are the ones who care.[1]

God loves *you and me, not because we are lovable, but because He is God.*

All of us had at least one person in the past who cared about us. Most of us have at least one person in the present who cares about us. If we are able to believe that other people really care about us, then why is it so hard to believe that God cares where we are—right here, right now?

I believe that part of the reason is that we don't know God as well as we know the humans who have cared about us and who care about us today. We do not know or do not believe that one word sums up God's character: love. God *loves* you and me, not because we are lovable, but because He is God. Take a minute to soak up this marvelous truth. God cares so much about where we are right now that He tries every day to get our attention.

A friend of mine has been going through a tough time lately. One of her children has been struggling, and she has been praying that God would break through and touch her child. Yesterday, as she was driving into work, she was feeling a great burden and she told God, "I'm giving this burden to you right now because it's too heavy for me to carry any longer." At a noon luncheon, as they were announcing a door prize for a getaway weekend, she thought to herself, *Wouldn't that be nice*, and immediately she heard her name called as the winner of the weekend away. She told me she believed that her name's being drawn from over 1,500 names of those attending reiterated to her that God cares where she is right now. You see, she was feeling lonely because she was sitting at a table with nine people she did not know; and God allowed her to win something for the first time in her life. Yesterday afternoon, after getting the care gram from God at the luncheon, she received a call telling her about a breakthrough in the life of her child!

This story has God's stamp all over it. If we think about it, every one of us has similar stories of God's care for us. God cares so much about where we are that He wants to show us in tangible ways. The very fact that you're reading this book is evidence that God cares about you and wants you to believe it. If we're looking for His hand in our present circumstances, we will see His care.

Psalm 147 tells us that God receives joy when we thank Him and praise Him in the midst of difficult circumstances. Would you, right now, stop reading and think about some things you might thank God for in the midst of your own circumstances? Pour your heart out to Him about your excess weight. Thank Him that He will receive praise and glory as He helps you lose the weight. Thank Him that He cares about where you are this very minute. Take some time and let God love you. Will you write a prayer of thanks to Him?

Dear Father,

God shows us every day how much He cares about where we are. Every day we have the opportunity to walk outside and watch the beautiful sunrise. The fact that we have a bed to sleep in and a roof over our heads is evidence of God's care. Just yesterday, as I was driving to work, I saw three deer standing by the road drinking from a pool of rainwater. I slowed my car and marveled at God's creation—these beautiful deer standing by the side of a busy thoroughfare. I thanked God that He cares about those deer and that He cares about me, too. He knows that I trust Him to write this book about losing weight while trying to do it myself. Looking at those trusting deer helped me acknowledge to God that I trust Him to reveal truths to me about the war to lose weight.

The biggest truth we must believe, if we are to lose weight and keep it off, is that God cares where we are. I will talk about the dailiness of life a little later in the book, but the dailiness of our lives is the biggest reason we forget how much God cares. If we could be transported to a beautiful place where no problems exist, we just know we could believe that God cares (sort of like my friend who thought, *Wouldn't that be nice*, at the luncheon). The reality is that getaways are few and far between. Life is full of problems every day, and your days are not very different from mine.

Choose to believe today that God cares where you are. Cast your burden of excess weight on Him today, believing that He cares for you and me and that He wants to help us not only to lose the weight but also to keep it off forever. Tell God that you're giving this burden to Him because you choose to believe He cares and that He wants to help you win the war.

PRAYER

Dear Father, help me believe that You care where I am today. Help me trust You to guide me each step of the way. I want to obey You so that I may offer You my life as a beautiful offering of usefulness and joy. In Jesus' name, amen.

CAROLE'S TRIPLE DARE JOURNAL

WEEK 7

Weight: 150 **Loss:** 1½ pounds

DAY 43 MONDAY, OCTOBER 21, 2002

Dailiness:
Time spent:
Accountability tip:

DAY 44 TUESDAY, OCTOBER 22, 2002

Dailiness: taught First Place class
Time spent: 3 hours
Accountability tip: Pat brought lunch for us.

DAY 45 WEDNESDAY, OCTOBER 23, 2002

Dailiness: California for Johnny's doctor's appointment
Time spent: all day
Accountability tip: didn't hold myself accountable–ate shrimp tempura at sushi restaurant

DAY 46 THURSDAY, OCTOBER 24, 2002

Dailiness: meetings at Gospel Light
Time spent: 5 hours
Accountability tip: ordered stir-fry chicken and veggies over rice–left half

DAY 47 FRIDAY, OCTOBER 25, 2002

Dailiness: breakfast with GL staff; videoed message for sales conference
Time spent: 3 hours
Accountability tip: ate all of Italian lunch (lacked accountability); three cannelloni with cheese and spinach, plus salad and bread; should have eaten only half of everything

DAY 48 SATURDAY, OCTOBER 26, 2002

Dailiness: came home from California
Time spent: all day
Accountability tip: no peanuts on plane, but ate Wheat Thins (10 grams of fat!)

DAY 49 SUNDAY, OCTOBER 27, 2002

Dailiness: tired–didn't go to church; unpacked, cleaned house, washed clothes
Time spent: all day
Accountability tip: don't feel good about tomorrow's weigh-in

CHAPTER 7

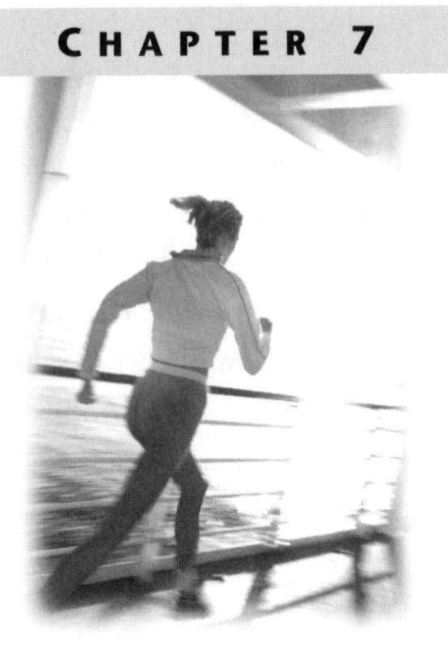

And even the very hairs of your head are all numbered.

MATTHEW 10:30

GOD CARES WHERE WE'RE GOING

Years ago my parents owned a house on Galveston Bay. Since the house was only one hour from Houston, where our entire family lived, often we would gather there in the summer. My brother-in-law, Roy, did not have a lot of hair. Because he was getting bald on top, he would let the hair on one side grow long enough to be able to part it low, comb it up and over the top and then smooth it into the hair on the other side. Once I realized what he was doing, I dearly loved pushing Roy off the pier at the bay to see this hair phenomenon as he emerged from the water. Roy would stand up in the water looking really strange, one side of his hair short and the other side long. He would always sputter, "Good gracious, Carole," all the way up the ladder, and we would all roar with laughter.

People tend to think that hair is primarily important to women, but hair has been important to both men and women since the beginning of time. As a woman, my greatest concern when I go somewhere is always my hair. Many of us talk about having a bad hair day as if this very fact were reason for the day to be ruined. Most of us spend more time getting our hair just right than anything else we do to get ready for the day. I believe that Jesus knew how much our hair means to us when He spoke the words recorded in Matthew 10:30. If God knows how many hairs are on our head, He must care greatly about us.

A friend told me once that the best way for her to get back on track was to go into "swimsuit therapy."

God not only cares about our hair, but He also cares about everything that concerns us. If we hate the way we look when we get dressed, God cares. If our clothes are too tight, God cares. If our feet hurt, God cares. God cares where we're going and desperately wants to help us look and feel good for the trip that He has planned for us. When we are overweight, we are less than enthusiastic about going places. We're uncomfortable squeezing into a booth at a restaurant. We worry about parties where we might have to sit in a lawn chair—what if it breaks? A swimsuit is out of the question. A friend told me once that the best way for her to get back on track was to go into "swimsuit therapy." She would go into the swimsuit department, pick out a bunch and proceed to try them on, one at a time. She said it was a surefire cure for the bingeing she had been doing, because she wasn't at all hungry when she left the store!

God cares where we're going, and He cares that we are unhappy about the way we look. Being overweight keeps us from wanting to get on board for the trip. In order to get back on track, we must believe not only that God cares where we're going but also that He plans for us to have a great time when we get there. Because God cares so much about where we're going, God put in every person's heart the desire to look good.

The most amazing thing about a trip is that we start getting excited the minute we finally leave home. The bags are packed, and even though we are just barely out of our driveway, we feel as though we're already there. The same thing happens when we decide to lose weight. Even though we might have a lot of weight to lose, we discover that after we lose even 10 pounds, our clothes start fitting a little better, and we begin to believe that we just might reach our goal.

God cares where we're going, but we'll never get there unless we agree to go on the journey with Him. Let's tell God right now that we want to go with Him on the journey to lose weight and get healthy. Tell Him that we are going to be like Abraham, who "obeyed and went, even though he did not know where he was going" (Heb. 11:8).

I became the full-time director of First Place in 1987. If I had known where God was going to take the First Place program from that day to this, I would have been scared to death. When I became the First Place director, we had 50 churches using the program. Today there are over 12,000 churches—in every state of the United States and in locations all over the world. If God had told me His plans, I would have responded that He had chosen the wrong person, because I didn't have the skills needed to make this happen.

Praise God that we don't know all the details when God asks us to join Him on the journey. God only wants us to believe, trust and obey Him today. As we do this, God is able to work mightily in our lives to accomplish His purposes. I have learned a valuable lesson as God has led me these last few years: It's not about us at all. It's all about God. We were created to bring honor and glory to God. When we stay focused on our present circumstances, we become overwhelmed and are unable to focus on a brighter future than the one we see today.

At Fitness Week one year, a lady who was obviously depressed attended. She was unhappy in her marriage and unhappy about her weight. She slept most of the day and stayed up most of the night on the

Internet. After just one week with us, she was nothing short of a miracle! She left Fitness Week with hope that her life could be different. Today she has lost weight and she is even helping lead a First Place class. She was able to catch the vision that God cared where she is going, and she grabbed hold of Him for the ride.

We must not start the journey based upon the emotion of the moment. If we sign up for the trip based on emotion, we'll be "letting our emotions dictate our actions, like letting the baggage do the driving."[1]

Deciding to take the journey with God to lose weight must be a conscious decision based on our belief that God knows and God cares where we've been, where we are and where we're going.

Prayer

Dear God, teach me to believe that You care where I'm going and that You want to help me get there. Help me trust You with the details. In Jesus' name, amen.

PART TWO

THE TRIPLE DARE

BELIEVE GOD, TRUST GOD, OBEY GOD

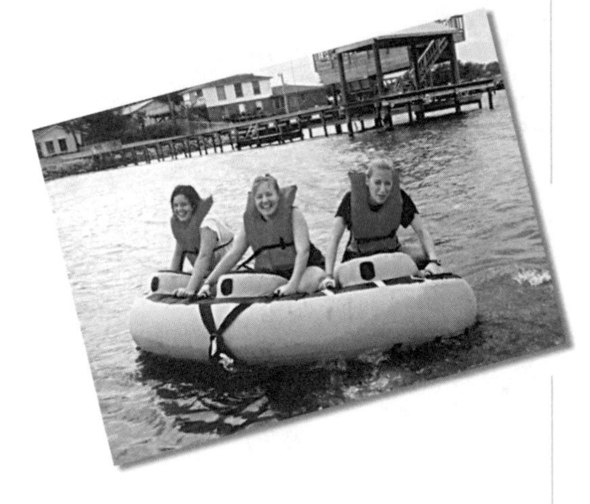

Carole's Triple Dare Journal

Week 8

Weight: 151 **Loss:** gained 1 pound

Day 50 Monday, October 28, 2002

Dailiness: back on track
Time spent: all day
Accountability tip: sobered by 1-pound gain

Day 51 Tuesday, October 29, 2002

Dailiness: led First Place class
Time spent: 3 hours
Accountability tip: brought vegetable soup from home for lunch

Day 52 Wednesday, October 30, 2002

Dailiness: staff lunch, radio interview, haircut, worked, went to see Mom
Time spent: 10 hours
Accountability tip: left cookie and chips at lunch; light turkey sandwich from Quizno's; grilled shrimp tacos for dinner—no fat

Day 53 Thursday, October 31, 2002

Dailiness: worked hard—three writing deadlines
Time spent: all day; got to work at 6:15 A.M.
Accountability tip: dinner—one meatball and 1 cup spaghetti

Day 54 Friday, November 1, 2002

Dailiness: started writing *Back on Track* preface and introduction
Time spent: 3 hours
Accountability tip: grilled chicken salad at Italian restaurant

Day 55 Saturday, November 2, 2002

Dailiness: wrote chapter 1
Time spent: 3 hours
Accountability tip: light chili and beans—no fat

Day 56 Sunday, November 3, 2002

Dailiness: wrote chapters 2 through 4
Time spent: 4 hours
Accountability tip: tuna poor boy—scooped out middle of poor-boy bun

CHAPTER 8

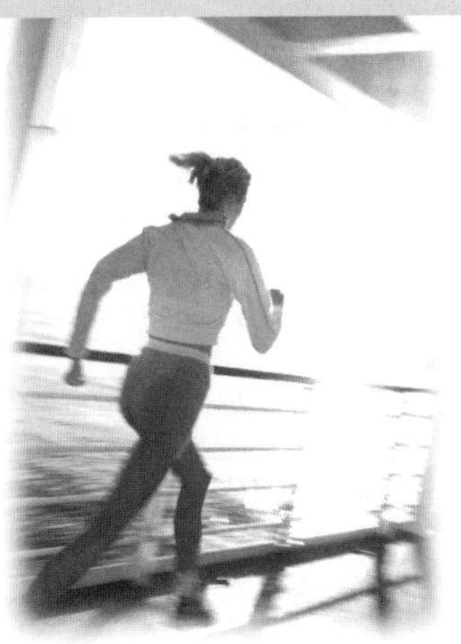

THE TRIPLE DARE

It was early morning on September 9, 2002, and I was curled up in my favorite living room chair having my quiet time. Little did I know that this would be a red-letter day for me, one I would never forget. It had been a rough year, starting the previous Thanksgiving night when our daughter Shari was struck and killed by a drunk driver. I was sitting there thanking and praising God for His faithfulness to me and my entire family. I was recounting in my mind all the ways God had shown us not only how much He knew where we had been this last year but also how much He cared.

As I told God how much I loved Him, I was suddenly struck with the realization of how little I really knew about loving God. I wrote in my prayer journal, "Lord, I want to love You more, but I don't have a clue how to do it. How can I show You how much I love You?" The Holy Spirit of God spoke one of our First Place memory verses very quietly into my ear. Let me paraphrase the verse for you, inserting my name so that you can get the full grasp of how I felt that day: "Carole, whoever has my commands and obeys them, she is the one who loves me. She who loves me will be loved by my Father, and I, too, will love her and show myself to her" (see John 14:21).

"Lord, I want to love You more, but I don't have a clue how to do it. How can I show You how much I love You?"

I learned that verse in 1981 in my very first session of First Place. Because I had memorized it many years earlier, God was able to bring it to my mind at the perfect time. I had quoted the verse many times, but for the very first time that morning the verse became personal to me—what you would call one of those aha moments. I wrote in my prayer journal, "Oh, that's it. You want me to obey you to show you how much I love you!" Well, duh; how do we as parents feel when our kids obey? We want to give them the world; just name it, it's theirs for the asking. As I mulled over the truth of the verse, the Holy Spirit spoke two words directly into my spirit: "It's time." I knew exactly what those words meant, because I was preparing to write this book. God told me that morning that He would show Himself to me and help me write the truth about losing weight if I would be willing to admit that I, too, had a problem losing weight. To do this I would need to share the struggles I have had getting back on track and then invite others to come along for the ride with me.

At first blush, I was humiliated. How could I, as the national director of First Place, share that I was having trouble in this area? God assured my heart that I would need to share not only that I had a struggle but also how big a struggle it had become. Whoa—this was really going to be hard. You see, when I joined First Place in March 1981, I was the biggest I had ever been in my life—133 pounds! If I had joined the program because I didn't want to be fat and 40, how was it going to look 21 years later to be even fatter and 60? God assured me that my pride was not bigger than He is and that I could do it, so I started to perk up and get a little bit excited about the journey.

When I got to work, I had an e-mail waiting for me from Kyle Duncan, publisher of Regal Books. Kyle told me how excited he was about the book and even offered to hire someone to help me write it if I needed help to meet the January deadline. As I read Kyle's e-mail, God confirmed in my heart and mind our early morning conversation. I joyously wrote back to Kyle that God had already given me the plan and that I wouldn't need any help writing the book. I didn't share with Kyle what the plan was, because I needed time to see if I could actually speak the words that at 60 years old I weighed 160 pounds! Well, God was faithful to show Himself to me as I agreed to be obedient. I started that very day and began to lose the weight.

On Saturday of that same eventful week, my granddaughter Cara and her college roommate, Katy, came to spend the weekend with us at Galveston Bay. We had purchased the Triple Dare, a water toy to pull behind our boat. This contraption is a 96-inch-long inflatable raft that has three raised sections on top, complete with handles to hold as you are pulled across the water behind a speeding boat. Cara and Katy were having a great time riding it. Johnny was driving the boat, and I was sitting in the swivel chair beside him watching the delight and horror on the faces of the girls as they were flung in and out of the wake at high speeds.

As I watched the girls, my heart ached at the losses these two girls had endured in their teenage years. Both had lost their moms during the past year. Katy had lost her mom in March 2001, during her senior year in high school, just three days after her eighteenth birthday. Cara had lost her mom (and we, our daughter) the following Thanksgiving. I felt this pang in my heart as I watched them on the outside positions of the Triple Dare, leaving the empty center section vacant. I so longed to be there for those two girls and to fill some of the vacancy in their hearts. I'm not a daring person at all, so it's almost incomprehensible that I asked Johnny that day, "Do you think I could ride that thing?" I guess God used my distress over their loss to spur me to be there for both of them and to take the dare to get on the Triple Dare myself. Johnny immediately said, "Well, I don't think you should!" After assuring him that I would let go if my body were hurting in any way, he agreed to let me try to ride the Triple Dare.

Johnny stopped the boat and I jumped into the water—which, I might add, was the easiest part of the entire ride. It was now time to somehow hoist my body up onto the Triple Dare. Since the raft was a good two feet high, this wasn't going to be easy. The girls did everything they could to help. Katy held my left leg up on the raft while Cara hoisted my backside upward. By the time I had positioned my 60-year-old body on top of the Triple Dare, I determined not to let go if it killed me! If I fell off in the middle of the bay, we would have to go through this ordeal again before I could get back to shore and get off.

The three of us had a fabulous ride and I was very proud of myself for being so daring—that is, until about 10:30 that night! My lower back was killing me and I told the girls, "I have really injured myself." I took some pain medicine and went to bed, being sure that I wouldn't be able to walk the next morning. I'm happy to tell you that when I awoke the next morning, after a night of hurting every time I turned over, I could walk. As I walked into my Sunday School class, I looked a little like a cowpoke who had ridden his horse for 16 hours straight! My thighs ached badly, and I was scheduled to make an announcement to the class about the class party at our home at the bay the next weekend. I walked as best I could to the podium and proceeded to tell the class about riding the Triple Dare the day before, challenging the entire class to do the same at the party. The only detail I left out about the ride was the fact of how badly I was hurting at that moment.

The next morning, I was in the same chair having my quiet time. The Lord spoke to my heart again and said, "Carole, this is the plan. You rode the Triple Dare because the challenge you are going to give all the people who desire to lose weight is this: They are to *believe God, trust God* and *obey God* for 16 weeks. That will be the Triple Dare. I want you to throw out the Triple Dare challenge to everyone you meet for the next few weeks."

I began doing just that and shared the plan the next day with my First Place group and another group that joined us for our halftime celebration. Two months before, when my coleader, Pat, and I planned our 13-week First Place session, we planned a halftime party for the halfway point of the session. Since it was football season, we decorated with a

The Lord said, "The challenge you are going to give all the people who desire to lose weight is this: They are to believe God, trust God *and* obey God *for 16 weeks. That will be the Triple Dare."*

halftime theme; and I was scheduled to speak to the two groups. You see, God knew and cared two months before as He helped us plan the entire session that I would be sharing the Triple Dare on that day.

That weekend I shared the plan at our First Place National Conference in Hattiesburg, Mississippi. On Sunday morning, after getting home late Saturday from Hattiesburg, I was driving to church and the Lord impressed my heart that I was to share the Triple Dare challenge with my Sunday School class. The only problem was that I wasn't teaching that Sunday. I told the Lord that I didn't think that would be possible, but if the teacher didn't show up, I would share the challenge. As I left my car to go into the church building, I picked up my Triple Dare notes along with my Bible. When our teacher came forward to teach the lesson, she did something unexpected. She called the class leadership team to the front and prayed for all of the leaders of the class. After she prayed, she issued a challenge to our class to volunteer to help the leadership team in some way. As she finished sharing about the need for the entire class to be involved in sharing the leadership load, I realized that this was what she had planned for the lesson that day—maybe she thought it would take longer than 15 minutes—and I watched her try to decide what we would do next. She asked if some might want to come and give a testimony for the remainder of our time together, and I knew in my heart that this was all part of God's plan for that morning. I got up from my chair, walked to the front and said, "God wants me to share something with the class this morning." I shared the plan with our Sunday School class that morning and then that night with another First Place class. I shared the Triple Dare one last time at our First Place Fitness Week on October 10, 2002. In one short month, God had allowed me to share the Triple Dare challenge to five groups, inviting each group to join me on the journey to lose weight. It was obvious to me that God knew and cared where I was going and that He allowed me to take the journey and to have it be like one big party every step of the way!

What about you? Will you take the Triple Dare to lose every pound you need to lose? Will you take the challenge to believe God, trust God and obey God for 16 weeks?

Prayer

Dear Father, this is one of the scariest things I've ever thought about. Do I dare to believe that You will show Yourself to me as You have done for Carole? Help me to have the courage to take the Triple Dare to believe, trust and obey You for 16 weeks. Help me to think only about today and not all the days ahead. In Jesus' name, amen.

WEEK 9

Weight: 149 **Loss:** 2 pounds—back on track!!!

DAY 57 MONDAY, NOVEMBER 4, 2002

Dailiness: wrote chapter 5
Time spent: 2 hours
Accountability tip: big lunch; scrambled-egg sandwich for dinner

DAY 58 TUESDAY, NOVEMBER 5, 2002

Dailiness: class victory celebration
Time spent: 2 hours
Accountability tip: salad bar—spinach instead of lettuce

DAY 59 WEDNESDAY, NOVEMBER 6, 2002

Dailiness: Inspire luncheon
Time spent: 2 hours
Accountability tip: left all three desserts!

DAY 60 THURSDAY, NOVEMBER 7, 2002

Dailiness: wrote chapter 6
Time spent: 2 hours
Accountability tip: lunch with Janice; split 8" vegetable pizza

DAY 61 FRIDAY, NOVEMBER 8, 2002

Dailiness: wrote chapters 7 and 8!!!
Time spent: 3 hours
Accountability tip: rice at cafeteria instead of roll

DAY 62 SATURDAY, NOVEMBER 9, 2002

Dailiness: A.M.—cleaned house; P.M.—church to see Yvonne receive Ruth Award in Shari's memory
Time spent: all day
Accountability tip:

DAY 63 SUNDAY, NOVEMBER 10, 2002

Dailiness: P.M.—cleaned house (Kay coming)
Time spent: 4 hours
Accountability tip: vegetable soup for dinner

CHAPTER 9

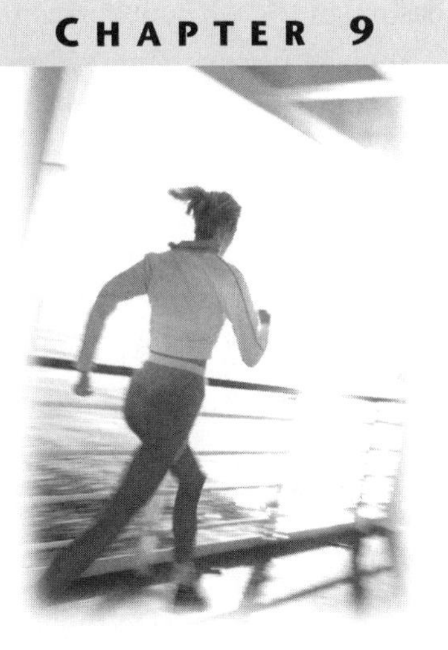

Without faith it is impossible to please God, because anyone who comes to him must believe that he exists and that he rewards those who earnestly seek him.

HEBREWS 11:6

BELIEVE GOD

BELIEF OF THE HEART

When God gave me His prescription to lose weight, it was a really simple prescription. God asked me—and those who would join me on this quest—to do three things. The first is to believe God.

Chapters 2 through 7 have endeavored to convince us that God knows and cares where we have been. If we've suffered, God knows it; and He cares about everything that has ever happened in our lives. God also knows and cares about where we are today. He knows if we are miserable about the weight we are carrying.

Most of us have chosen to read this book because we are carrying around physical weight. The truth of the matter is that when our bodies are overweight, we are carrying around more than the excess pounds: we are carrying excess weight in our hearts. Our heart is the seat of our mind, will and emotions; and our emotions play a huge role in our own personal battle of the bulge. The Bible has much to say about carrying excess weight in our hearts. Romans 10:10 says, "It is with your heart that you believe and are justified."

When our bodies are overweight, we are carrying around more than the excess pounds: we are carrying excess weight in our hearts.

We desperately want to believe that God knows and cares about where we are today. Even if we believe it, it may not do anything to move us off dead center to lose the pounds we desperately want to lose. You see, unless we begin believing that God cares where we are right now and that He has the power to help us make the needed changes to lose weight, we will never lose weight and keep it off forever.

Our minds and bodies will cooperate with what our hearts believe about God's ability to help us lose all the weight we need to lose. In our heart of hearts, do we really believe that God knows and cares where we are today? If we have accepted the free gift of salvation, our spirits are secure forever. The real problem is convincing our hearts that God really knows and cares and wants to help us here and now. The verse used at the beginning of this chapter says that we must believe that God exists and that He rewards those who earnestly seek Him. Unless our hearts and minds are filled with the truth found only in the Bible, God's Holy Word, we will continue to fail at losing weight.

Do we believe that God wants to reward us with a healthy body that weighs the right amount and is able to perform the daily tasks God has for us to do? Our heart is the real culprit when it comes to believing God.

Because our heart is damaged by the world's belief system, we must learn to believe that God wants to reward us with weight loss and good health as we earnestly seek Him. If we don't believe God in our hearts, we are destined to fail at keeping the weight off after we lose it. Our mind already knows enough to lose weight and to keep it off forever. Our emotions are the villain when it comes to being successful in this area of our lives.

Attacks on the Heart

As I sat in my chair on September 9 and reflected on the last 12 years, I realized that my heart had been bombarded with all kinds of physical and emotional difficulties. I had endured physical injuries, surgeries and physical therapy on numerous occasions. I had given up being diligent when it came to my weight and had let the pounds creep up and up until I found myself being 60 years old, directing a national weight-loss program and weighing 160 pounds. As I share my own personal struggle to believe in my heart of hearts that my weight problems are important enough to God for Him to want to help me, it is my prayer that each of you who reads this book makes the choice to believe in your heart that God wants to do the same for you.

In September 1991, I started training for the Houston marathon. I was celebrating my fiftieth birthday on January 2, 1992, and I really wanted to enter a second half-century of living by running a marathon. Having never run over six miles at one time, I knew that if I were to finish the 26.2-mile run, I would need to train diligently. Since the race is always held in January, I believed that I could be ready for it in four months. I even planned to start a marathon training program after I worked up to being able to consistently run 30 miles per week. From previous study, I knew not to add more than 10 percent per week to my running base; but I was anxious to start the marathon training program, so I pushed myself beyond what I knew was safe and sound. In three short weeks I went from running 10 to 12 miles per week to running 30 miles per week. In doing this, I went beyond what I knew was safe training and I tore the cartilage in my right knee. As I look back, the hurt in my heart about not being able to run much anymore was the beginning of my real problem with weight gain.

I needed to lose 20 pounds when I joined First Place in 1981. I had lost the same 20 pounds more than a few times, but it was always easy for me to lose it once I got back on track. Staying on track was much easier for me after I started jogging in 1984. Jogging was something I could do every day, and I could do it alone. I could meet my own personal goals and not worry about what someone else did, because I ran for the sheer love of running. I absolutely loved how running made me feel. After I finished my morning run, I was pumped and ready to meet the day. Running had turned me from a person who resisted structure and plans to one who actually planned my day as I ran. I can easily see today how not being able to run any longer had a huge effect on my emotions and why I allowed my weight to escalate over the next 10 to 12 years. The injury to my right knee was only the beginning of my physical trials, and emotional trials were not far behind either. Let me list them for you:

The Reality—Physical

March 1994	Bone spur in neck—three weeks in bed/physical therapy.
October 1994	Ankle injury in the Smokies—six weeks in boot and crutches.
February 1997	Fell at restaurant/wet floor—tore rotator cuff in both shoulders and cartilage in both knees.
June 1997	Right-shoulder surgery—six weeks physical therapy.
May 1998	Ear surgery—hole in eardrum.
August 1998	Left-shoulder surgery—six weeks physical therapy.
November 1999	Right-knee surgery—six weeks physical therapy.

The Reality—Emotional

September 1994	My sister Glenda died of major stroke three weeks after her sixtieth birthday—lost my only sibling.

September 1995	Sister-in-law, Donna, died—lost one of my best friends of 35 years and my interior decorator.
October 1997	Son, John's, home burned—his family of five moved into our home with nothing but the clothes on their backs.
October 1997	Husband, Johnny, was diagnosed with stage 4 prostate cancer that had spread to his pelvic bones.
October 1997	Monumental move to Galveston Bay after 55 years of living in Houston—two hour commute to work.
November 1999	Moved my 87-year-old mom into our home—became full-time caregiver.
November 2001	39-year-old daughter, Shari, killed by a drunk driver on Thanksgiving night—leaving her husband, Jeff, without his wife and her three teenage daughters without their mother. Our son, John, and daughter Lisa lost their sister; and Johnny and I lost our child.
June 2002	Forced to move Mom to personal care home—I visited her on my way home from work.
October 2002	Mom in hospital for three weeks to insert feeding tube—decisions regarding care.
November 2002	Mom pulled out feeding tube. Taken by ambulance to hospital. Spent 12 hours holding her hands so that she wouldn't hurt herself.

I relate these incidents in my own life to jog your memory of your own past. You might even want to get a piece of paper and write down some of the things that have kept you from believing that God wants to help you lose weight and to keep it off. We all have events in our lives—some that are small, frustrating and distracting and some that are traumatic—that can discourage us from trusting God. Will we allow the events of our daily lives to make us bitter or better? Will we become a victim or victor? Will we be overcome or will we be an overcomer? Will we choose to believe that God knows and cares and wants to help us succeed?

After I asked my assistant, Pat, to pull these dates and events together for me, I was shocked that so much had happened in 10 short years.

God loves His kids.

I say "10 short years" because the time has flown by rapidly and it has been a time of great joy and growth in the Lord. One of my favorite verses this past year, since losing Shari, has been, "I would have despaired unless I had believed that I would see the goodness of the LORD in the land of the living" (Ps. 27:13, *NASB*). God has not failed me one time during the last 10 years. Each trial has shown me that God is faithful and that He can be believed.

Rivers of Joy

While enduring physical and emotional pain during those years, I have experienced rivers of joy. God gave us the most wonderful publisher, Regal Books, in 2000, and we have been blessed "exceeding abundantly beyond all that we ask or think" (Eph. 3:20, *NASB*). Our First Place materials are exactly what we had dreamed they would become when we were in the throes of material revisions.

I have had three books published, and I am joyously writing this fourth book with God's help. God has allowed Johnny and me to live in a home for the last five years where we can lie in bed and watch the sun rise over Galveston Bay. We have a wonderful family and extended family—we love each other and want to be together whenever we have the opportunity. I could go on and on, enumerating the blessings of God to me, given not only the last 10 years but given every year since I accepted Jesus at the age of 12.

God knows and cares and can be believed because He is good. Jesus sticks closer than a brother, and God is the most loving Father we could ever imagine. Why not take a few minutes right now and list some of the many blessings in your own life? I promise that the blessings list will always be longer than the difficulties list. You know why? Because our God loves His kids. When we belong to the family of God, we can be assured that if we will believe, trust and obey Him the best we know how, He will come in and work miracles in and through us.

The Choice to Believe

Make the conscious choice to believe God with me today. Believe that God wants to help us lose all the weight we need to lose. Believe that God will give us strength when we are weak, if we will only ask Him. Believe that God has a wonderful future planned for us. Choose to believe in order to receive. The Bible tells a story in the ninth chapter of Mark about a man who came to Jesus, asking for healing for his son. Jesus told the man, "Everything is possible for him who believes." The man answered, "I do believe; help me overcome my unbelief" (vv. 23-24). Won't you tell Jesus those same words right now? If you know Jesus, you have believed that He has the power to come in and change your life. Ask Him to help you overcome your unbelief about His wanting to help you lose weight and keep it off forever.

Prayer

Dear Lord, I want to believe that You know and care about everything that concerns me today. Help my unbelief. Teach me what it means to have a Father who knows and cares and who can fix my brokenness. In Jesus' name, amen.

WEEK 10

Weight: 148½ **Loss:** ½ pound

DAY 64 MONDAY, NOVEMBER 11, 2002

Dailiness: wrote chapter 9
Time spent: 3 hours
Accountability tip: split lunch

DAY 65 TUESDAY, NOVEMBER 12, 2002

Dailiness: picked up Kay at airport
Time spent: 2 hours
Accountability tip: vegetable soup before Beth's Bible study

DAY 66 WEDNESDAY, NOVEMBER 13, 2002

Dailiness: planning for 2003
Time spent: 8 hours
Accountability tip: cafeteria–good choices

DAY 67 THURSDAY, NOVEMBER 14, 2002

Dailiness: planning
Time spent: 8 hours
Accountability tip: Vietnamese–chicken with rice

DAY 68 FRIDAY, NOVEMBER 15, 2002

Dailiness: shopped after work with Kay
Time spent: 3 hours
Accountability tip: cereal for dinner

DAY 69 SATURDAY, NOVEMBER 16, 2002

Dailiness: shopped with Kay
Time spent: 6 hours
Accountability tip: egg on toast for dinner

DAY 70 SUNDAY, NOVEMBER 17, 2002

Dailiness: went to church
Time spent: 6 hours
Accountability tip: split lunch; got into cookies the last two weeks

CHAPTER 10

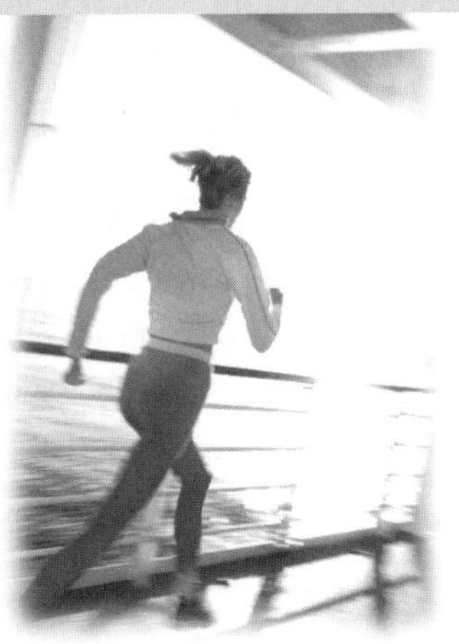

> *Those who know your name will trust in you, for you, LORD, have never forsaken those who seek you.*
>
> PSALM 9:10

TRUST GOD

CUT THE ROPE

I heard a story about a mountain climber who wanted to climb the highest mountain. He began his adventure after many years of preparation; but since he wanted the glory just for himself, he decided to climb the mountain alone. He started to climb, and it began to get very late; but instead of preparing his tent to camp, he kept climbing until it got very dark.

The night felt heavy in the heights of the mountain, and the man could not see anything. All was black—with zero visibility because clouds covered the moon and the stars. As he was climbing, only a few feet away from the top of the mountain, he slipped and fell over the edge of the mountain, falling at a great speed. The climber could only see black spots as he went down and felt the terrible sensation of being sucked by gravity. He kept falling, and in those moments of great fear, his life flashed before him.

He was thinking now of how close death was getting, when all of a sudden he felt the rope that was tied to his waist pull him very hard. His body was hanging in the air—only the rope was holding him—and in that moment of stillness, he had no other choice but to scream, "Help me, God!"

All of a sudden, a deep voice coming from the sky answered, "What do you want me to do?" The man cried out, "Save me, God!" God answered, "Do you really think I can save you?" "Of course I believe You can," the man shouted. God said, "Then cut the rope." There was a moment of silence. The man decided to hang on to the rope with all his strength.

"Do you really think I can save you?" God said. "Then cut the rope."

The rescue team tells that the next day a climber was found dead and frozen—his body hanging from a rope. His hands were holding tight to the rope—only 10 feet above the ground.

This is a powerful story that makes each of us give serious thought to whether we trust God enough to cut the rope that is holding us today. Our rope might be the rope of unbelief that God knows, cares and wants to help us. Our rope might be the rope of bitterness, anger, hopelessness or grief about events of our past or present circumstances.

Look over the events of your own life. What ropes are you hanging on to and refusing to cut? Until you cut them, God is unable to come in and set you free.

Afraid to Trust

I have many women friends who have survived tragic circumstances of sexual, physical, emotional and verbal abuse. Many of these women no longer live in an abusive relationship. They have husbands and children who love them. Others have chosen mates who are abusive, because they still feel unworthy of love. I have watched marriages disintegrate and children become distant, and even abusive, because of the dysfunction of the past that is brought into the present. These women have battled being overweight for most of their lives. They have lost weight time and again, only to gain it all back, plus some.

Without exception, whether these women have a good marriage, a bad marriage or multiple marriages or have never been married at all, they have one thing in common: a problem trusting God. They can trust God for their spouse, their children and their friends and for help in so many areas of their lives, but not that God cares enough about them personally to want to help them lose weight and become the vibrant Christians they desperately want to be. They have a real problem believing and trusting that God has a wonderful future planned especially for them. Many times the lack of trust comes from not being able to trust their earthly parents. Because our earthly parents model God to us, any kind of troubled childhood can cause us not to be able to trust God.

A few years ago while attending a staff retreat, I had an experience of what it must feel like for those who are afraid to trust. Our staff went through a ropes course as a team-building exercise. One of the maneuvers was to help each other climb a very tall wall. After we all got to the top of the wall, our team took turns standing on either side of an opening, which was open all the way to the ground below. All but one member of the team locked arms across the opening; the other member would stand at the top of the wall, back turned to the team, and would fall backward into their arms.

When it was my turn to fall from the ledge, I believed that I wouldn't fall to the ground, because I had been part of the group catching the others as they fell. I had watched others fall into our arms, which were locked tightly together, and no one had been hurt. The problem came when I had to turn around backward and hurl my own body into space before I reached their safe arms. It was so hard to let go that I thought the man helping me literally would have to push me backward. The man kept encouraging me gently that I could do it and that I should just let go and fall. By the time I finally let go, I was embarrassed at the length of time I had been standing on that ledge.

As I fell backward and felt the comfort of all those arms catching my body, I was instantly aware that the fear I had felt must be the same kind of fear that keeps so many from trusting God. We know in our heads that God can be trusted, but our hearts seem unable to muster up the courage to let go and trust Him. What if He drops us? What if we fail?

Our Trustworthy God

I have learned that God can be trusted with my life. He has never let me down—not one time—when I have trusted Him with a problem. Back in 1984, when Johnny lost his business and we were broke—with a son still in college—God came through in might and power as we clung to Him and trusted Him to help. God taught me through that trial that all the material things of this world are not that important. He has the power to give us back those material things because He knows and cares about His kids.

Another thing God showed me during this painful time was that, more than anything, He wanted a relationship with me that was close and personal. He wanted me to come to Him, admitting that I had made a mess of my life and that I needed help to get it back together. Because God is a loving Father, He not only helped me as I sought Him, but He also taught me lessons that I couldn't have learned any other way.

I do not believe that suffering is ever God's intention for our lives. I do believe, however, that suffering and trouble are part of life because we live in a fallen world. God has taught me through every trial I have gone through that He always uses our suffering for His glory and for our good. This is one of God's promises to His children found in Romans 8:28. If we know Christ, all of our trials and tribulations will work together for good. When we refuse to trust Him as we walk through those dark times, a terrible thing happens: we start believing that God cannot be trusted, because we feel so alone. We feel alone because we sometimes run away from God instead of straight into His arms, as He intended.

In September, one of our cats died. On my drive to work, Johnny called me and asked if I had seen the cat the night before or that morning when I left the house. I told him that I hadn't seen her; he said that when it got light, he would go out and look for her. He found her body down on the rocks by the water where someone had thrown her. He lovingly picked her up, carried her home and buried her. Later that day he wrote a story about her; I would like you to read it. I haven't changed one word, but I did title his story "Trust." See if you see yourself as you read Johnny's story.

Trust

Tuesday, September 17, 2002

I buried our cat, Sneaky, today. Sneaky came into our lives when we moved to the bay in October 1997. We named her Sneaky not because she was conniving but because she was sneaky in a survival way: always wary and sneaking around.

Sneaky slept in our garage, and when I first heard her knock something over, I looked out the kitchen door that opened into our garage. Sneaky and I made eye contact and she quickly disappeared through a hole in the back of the garage. It was obvious that at no time in her life did she have any reason to trust or have faith in any human being.

It took several months of putting out food for her, slowly moving the dish from the back of the garage to finally having her eat from the dish as it sat on the kitchen floor. She put her trust in us and we never let her down. Sometimes she would not come home for two or three days, but she always reappeared.

Sneaky could not see or hear very well, but she could recognize cars. When our family came to visit and there were strange cars in the driveway, she would stay in the garage and not come into the house to eat until everyone was gone.

Regardless of what had happened in Sneaky's early life and whatever abuse she had suffered, she knew she was loved and welcome in our home. When she would disappear every evening, we would look down the driveway the next morning to see if she was returning again. We always felt relieved when we saw her.

It is the same with God. Regardless of our past, whether the way we treated people or the way we were treated, God takes us back and is relieved when we reappear.

We will miss Sneaky. I learned so much from her. She was a survivor.

John Lewis
Cancer survivor for 5 years

A dear friend of mine is a survivor of sexual, verbal and emotional abuse. She has huge trust issues because of all she has suffered. During the time I was walking with her through her healing journey, she made a statement that I will never forget: "People only get one chance with me. If they let me down or hurt me, they don't get a second chance to do it again."

Each time we begin again, God welcomes us with open arms of love. He is a loving heavenly Father who can be trusted.

I watched this statement play out in her life over and over again, even though it hurt me each time it happened. I believe that the reason she didn't trust others was because she didn't believe that God could be trusted. If she couldn't trust God, then she certainly couldn't trust a human who let her down or hurt her.

Aren't we glad that our God doesn't treat us this way? What if the next time we mess up, God said, "Well, this is one time too many. You have hurt

Me for the last time. Don't come back and ask Me to forgive you; this is your last chance with Me."

Remember, God doesn't love like we do. Our love for others is sometimes conditional, and we make the rules about whom we will love and how much we will love. God's love for us is unconditional and knows no limits. It doesn't matter at all to God that we have failed so many times to lose weight. Each time we begin again, God welcomes us with open arms of love. He is a loving heavenly Father who can be trusted.

The Choice to Trust

If you are a survivor of any kind of abuse, your biggest hurdle in taking the Triple Dare will be believing God, and trusting Him will be the next. Each time fear fills your heart, tell God out loud, "I trust You to take care of me." Each time our enemy, the devil, tells you that you should have never taken this challenge and that you won't make it, just give his message to God and ask God to answer it for you.

Others who read this book have had no abuse in their past. The reality is that any of us who struggle with being overweight have trouble believing that God can and will help us if we will only cooperate with Him. Trusting God is easy when times are good, but trusting God when life is chaotic is hard. Because we don't feel His presence, we think He's not there for us.

Trusting God involves running to Him, much like a child who has a cut comes running into the house, screaming for help. The child knows that if he or she can just get to Mama, help is on the way. The child trusts that as soon as the blood is washed off and a Band-Aid is applied to the cut, life will be better. The child has the full assurance that help will come from his or her earthly parent. The Bible says in Matthew 7:11, "If you, then, though you are evil, know how to give good gifts to your children, how much more will your Father in heaven give good gifts to those who ask Him!" God is our heavenly Father, and He can be trusted.

Believing and trusting God are the first steps in losing weight; obeying God is next. Obeying God involves work on our part, but God promises to give us the strength to obey when we ask for it. Friends, coworkers and family can encourage us along the way, too. Our job is to do the hard work of choosing healthy foods to eat and putting on our walking shoes to go for a daily walk.

Prayer

Dear Father, I want to trust You with my whole heart. I want to run to You, screaming about the shape of my body. I am heartsick about the way I look and feel. Help me learn what it means to believe You and to trust You to help me change. In Jesus' name, amen.

WEEK 11

Weight: 148 **Loss:** ½ pound

DAY 71 MONDAY, NOVEMBER 18, 2002

Dailiness: came into office at 6 A.M. to write; ended up reading e-mails—ugh!
Time spent: 2 hours
Accountability tip: don't read e-mails first!!

DAY 72 TUESDAY, NOVEMBER 19, 2002

Dailiness: spoke for holiday First Place class
Time spent: 3 hours, with preparation time
Accountability tip: split baked potato—ranch dressing on top

DAY 73 WEDNESDAY, NOVEMBER 20, 2002

Dailiness: came in at 6 A.M. to write
Time spent: 3 hours
Accountability tip: vegetable lunch at cafeteria

DAY 74 THURSDAY, NOVEMBER 21, 2002

Dailiness: cleaned house after work
Time spent: 3 hours
Accountability tip: ate some of Johnny's steak—ordered extra salad

DAY 75 FRIDAY, NOVEMBER 22, 2002

Dailiness: wrote chapter 10
Time spent: 3 hours
Accountability tip: saved soup and bread from lunch

DAY 76 SATURDAY, NOVEMBER 23, 2002

Dailiness: shopping with daughter Lisa and three grandkids
Time spent: 9 hours
Accountability tip: grazed in SAM'S CLUB; no dinner 'til midnight—not good

DAY 77 SUNDAY, NOVEMBER 24, 2002

Dailiness: three grandkids got Blizzards (didn't get one)
Time spent: 30 minutes
Accountability tip: no desserts

CHAPTER 11

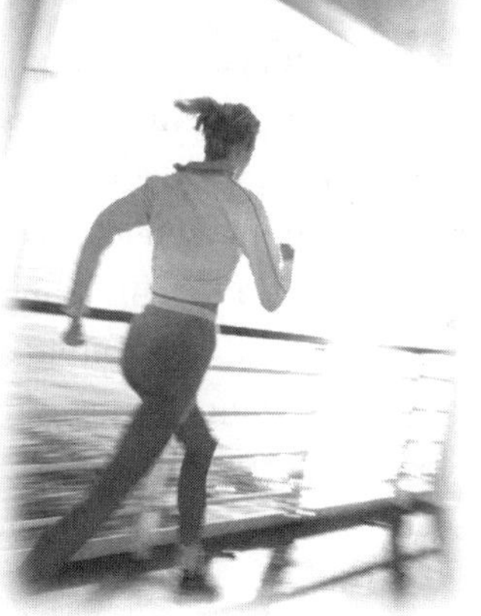

> *Whoever has my commands and obeys them, he is the one who loves me. He who loves me will be loved by my Father, and I too will love him and show myself to him.*
>
> JOHN 14:21

OBEY GOD

THE BOWSER BOYS

We have two one-year-old golden retrievers, Beau and Major.

Our daughter Shari and her husband, Jeff, received a golden retriever puppy as a wedding gift from one of Shari's favorite teachers, who raised this breed. Shari and Jeff had Goldie for many years, and after Goldie died they always had one or two golden retrievers in their family. This is a gentle breed—great with children—so at the time of Shari's death, their family had two of these dogs, and the female was going to have puppies.

While I was in Canada in February 2002, our oldest granddaughter, Cara, called Johnny and said—as only a granddaughter can say—"Dampi, the most beautiful of all the puppies is Beau. I was going to take Beau to Texas A&M next semester, and we were going to get an apartment. Katy's dad won't let her move to an apartment, so we will have to stay in the dorm. Do you think you and Mimi might take Beau?" Johnny temporarily took leave of his senses and said yes; so when I got home, Beau was on his way to the bay to live with us.

The first night we put paper all over the floor and confined him to one big room. The next morning not only had Beau done his business on and off the paper, but he also had systematically torn the paper to shreds. Beau also barked, howled and scratched the door all night.

The next night after a First Place council meeting, I bought a huge kennel and placed Beau inside with a nice, soft towel and a couple of toys. As we were trying to go to sleep, Beau was howling and barking intermittently; so we got up, put Beau in a closet, shut the door and then shut the door of the room he was in and every door between Beau and our bedroom in order to be able to get any sleep at all.

A few days into this routine, I was talking with Jeff, who had just one puppy left. I was telling Jeff about Beau's nonstop barking, scratching and howling; and Jeff said, "You know, Carole, it might be easier with two dogs, because they will keep each other company." I immediately took leave of my own senses and heard myself saying, "That makes sense." So that weekend Major arrived.

As the dogs have grown older, they've gained more and more weight, until now each of them weighs over 100 pounds. And not only are they beautiful and lovable, but they are also wild.

In October of that same year, my mom was in the hospital. After a particularly harrowing day with the dogs, whom we affectionately call the Bowser Boys, Johnny came to the hospital to visit Mom and to sit with me. That day, while opening the gate of the pen to feed the dogs, Beau had plowed right over Johnny, knocking him into the side of a flagstone planter box. He already had cuts on his arms—in various stages of healing—from the dogs jumping up on him, and now a huge scrape on his leg was added. The situation was summed up perfectly when a nurse came into the hospital room and said to Johnny, "Oh my goodness, have you been in a wreck?"

After the nurse left the room, Johnny said to me, "We have to do something about the dogs. Either we hire a trainer or we have to give them away. They are going to kill one or both of us if we don't."

The week before, we had been taking them from the pier back to their pen on a leash, and I was leading Major. Actually, Major was leading me and literally dragged me across the yard on my face, because Beau, who was in the lead, took off running and Major instinctively followed. One of our neighbors witnessed the episode and, knowing Johnny has cancer, took pity on us. Every day for about three days, Chuck showed up at 6:30 A.M. and 6:30 P.M. and walked each of those dogs, for 20 minutes at a time, trying to teach them to obey. Now, you need to understand, Chuck had hired a trainer for his two labs, so this was a genuine act of love and compassion for him to come to our rescue. Beau and Major were actually a little better when Beau plowed Johnny down, but the fact remained that they were huge by this time.

I had to leave for Fitness Week while Mom was still in the hospital. Johnny and I had decided that after all the time and money we had already invested in the dogs, we would hire a trainer and see if he might be able to teach them to obey. The results were astounding. After just one session, Johnny called me and said, "You are not going to believe the way the Bowser Boys behave for this guy. He already has them sitting when he gives the command. After just one lesson, they are so much better." Well, the trainer came 10 times and the Boys learned to sit, stay and heel.

Even though the Bowser Boys had improved, there were still a few more hurdles, which required even more money to be spent. You see, they still wanted to leave our fenced yard, go around the ends of the fence and get on the rocks leading to the water in order to escape. To ensure their safety, we were forced to extend the fence further down to the water on both sides so that they couldn't get out and be hurt. Even this last week, we had to buy more cyclone fencing and place it on the rocks so that the dogs wouldn't want to walk across and escape.

Lessons Learned from the Boys

You might be wondering why I spent so much time talking about these two dogs in relation to losing weight and obeying God. Let me assure you, God has used our Bowser Boys to teach me more about obedience than I ever cared to know.

One big lesson I have learned is that all of us have boundaries, and if we stay inside those boundaries, we are safe and secure. We have an acre of land, with 160 feet of waterfront. Those two dogs should be elated

God has used our Bowser Boys to teach me more about obedience than I ever cared to know.

living in this beautiful place, because they have the opportunity to get in the water and swim whenever they like—and golden retrievers love water. They have a huge yard where they can run and play, with shady areas to rest when they get hot and tired, and they have food and water available all the time. Yet their greatest desire is to leave the safe boundaries of our yard and run toward a busy intersection where many neighborhood dogs have been killed.

Most domesticated animals can be taught to obey. By reinforcing commands time after time, the animal learns to submit to its owner's voice. There is no prerequisite that the animal has to want to obey. But God created us higher than the animals. He created us in His own image, giving us free will and the right to choose to obey Him. We can learn obedience by submitting to Christ's control in our lives. He is willing and waiting to take charge and help us succeed, but we must make the choice to obey. The problem in losing weight is that we must bring our flesh under submission to God. Paul says in 1 Corinthians 9:27, "No, I beat my body and make it my slave," indicating that we have a vital role in this area of obeying God. We must choose each day to eat healthy food instead of the foods that ultimately keep us defeated, overweight and unfit.

As I've observed the bizarre behavior of Beau and Major, God has taught me that many of us remind Him a lot of those two Bowser Boys. God gave us the most beautiful home to live in called Earth. We can enjoy gorgeous sunrises and sunsets. We have the opportunity to walk through parks and around lakes, basking in the beauty that our God created especially for our pleasure. Instead, we sit for mindless hours in front of our television sets or computers, burning very few calories.

We have a vast array of healthy foods at our disposal. We have grocery stores overflowing with beautiful fruits and vegetables, an endless variety of whole grains and every kind of lean meat to eat. We can eat to our fill from these kinds of foods and not have a problem losing weight. Most of us have legs that are strong, and we can take long walks in beautiful surroundings. What do we do instead? We eat every kind of unhealthy food available to us. We eat these foods fried and supersized; then we top off the meal with a high-calorie dessert. While consuming huge amounts of calories, we grouse endlessly about how hard it is to lose weight.

Just like Johnny and I want to shower those Bowser Boys with love and the opportunity for enjoyment, so God wants to shower us with His love and give us everything we desire, if we will only obey Him. God wants to give us long, healthy, useful lives of service to Him; but we refuse to obey because we want the temporary pleasures so readily available to us. Just like God gave Adam and Eve all kinds of trees in the Garden of Eden that were pleasing to look at and to eat, God will provide every kind of good food for us—foods so endless in variety that we'll never get tired or bored with the choices. And just like Adam and Eve were not allowed to eat from one tree in the Garden for their own good, there are some foods that we need to stay away from for our own good—foods that will harm our bodies, foods that will keep up from the plans He has for our lives.

The Choice to Obey

First Place, the program I direct, is a comprehensive health program. The program is complete with food lists, Bible studies, wellness worksheets, commitment records and exercise plans. First Place groups provide accountability and support. As members of First Place we know that when we do the plan, the plan works. Why is it, then, that even with these fabulous tools, those of us in First Place have trouble losing weight and keeping it off?

The problem lies in the fact that we refuse to believe God, trust God or obey God in the area of our eating and exercise. When Adam and Eve gave in to the temptation that was offered by Satan that fateful day in the Garden—to eat from the tree of the knowledge of good and evil—sin entered the human race. That is the same sin we deal with on a daily basis. Those of us who are Christians have the very power of Christ living inside of us, ready to help us accomplish God's perfect will for our lives. When we believe that God's way is best and we trust God to help us, it then becomes our responsibility to obey God as He shows how to lose the weight we want to lose.

Joseph Stowell said it so well:

> Loving God and living to experience the mismanaged passion of our souls are mutually exclusive. But when we surrender in love to Him, He helps us manage our passions and their relationship to the people and the things that surround us. Choosing to love God with our passions keeps us within safe boundaries and opens up the world of all that is pleasurably legitimate yet without shame and regret. If we live to experience the urges of our passions apart from the guiding hand of God, our love for Him is only a charade. We must remember that for the believer every choice to fulfill our own wants and needs apart from God inevitably ends in sorrow and sin. "The one who sows to please his sinful nature, from that nature will reap destruction" (Galatians 6:8).[1]

I am now in week 11 of the Triple Dare to believe God, trust God and obey God; and I must say, this is the easiest time I have ever had losing weight. I haven't worried about planning meals or about what I will eat, like in times past. So far, I have relaxed in the arms of my Savior, Jesus Christ, and I've allowed Him to show me the way to go almost every day. Losing weight is really not hard. Everyone who reads this book has proven this many times. The real problem is gaining weight, because most of us seem destined to gain back the weight we lose—plus a few more pounds each time. God is gently teaching me that His way works. If I will obey a few simple commands, not only will He help me lose this excess weight I have accumulated, but He will help me keep it off forever. God wants to do the same for you. The question is, Will you obey?

The other day, we were outside with the Bowser Boys. One gate wasn't shut securely and Major got out. As Johnny opened the gate to go after Major, Beau shot past him and went running down the street to catch up with Major. After I got their leashes, we finally got them back into the yard and into their pen. Later that night, Johnny said to me, "You know, there are two words that I always say. I say it about the dogs all the time." "What two words?" I asked. Johnny replied, "'That's it!' Every time the dogs get out, I say, 'That's it!' They're staying in the pen from now on. I used to say it to the kids. 'That's it! Give me the car keys.' 'That's it! You're grounded.'" He went on to say that he didn't mean it then and he doesn't mean it now.

I started thinking about what Johnny said and realized how grateful I am that God never says that to you or me. God has never once said to me, "That's it!" Many times I have deserved that kind of response, but it has never happened—not once. God has shown me only unconditional love, grace and mercy. He welcomes me back each time I do something wrong or don't do something right.

I know that God smiles when we are obedient, just like Johnny and I smile when the Bowser Boys are good. I'm sure it saddens God when we disobey and when we just don't get it, but He never becomes exasperated and says, "That's it!" God knows us inside and out. He knows that, without His power, we are not capable of doing much right.

Aren't we glad that God created us with a will, to choose between right and wrong? Without the option to make wrong choices, our right choices wouldn't mean much. God wants to give us everything that He has planned to give us from the foundation of the world—if we would only obey. Will we do it?

Prayer

Dear Lord, obeying You will be the hardest part of the Triple Dare—I had just thought it would be hard to believe and trust You. To obey You will mean that I quit eating the comfort foods I love. It will mean that I take a walk when I would rather watch television. Help me to obey You. Change my wants and desires so that they line up with Your will for my life. In Jesus' name, amen.

Carole's Triple Dare Journal

Week 12

Weight: 148 **Loss:** stayed same

Day 78 Monday, November 25, 2002

Dailiness: with Mom in hospital
Time spent: 8 hours
Accountability tip: keeping Commitment Record—will lose weight next Monday!

Day 79 Tuesday, November 26, 2002

Dailiness: worked on book
Time spent: 3 hours
Accountability tip: cafeteria—good choices

Day 80 Wednesday, November 27, 2002

Dailiness: met with reporter for *Houston Chronicle* article
Time spent: 3 hours
Accountability tip: vegetable soup and crackers for dinner; kids ate pizza

Day 81 Thursday, November 28, 2002

Dailiness: Thanksgiving with family
Time spent: all day
Accountability tip: ate healthily, no dessert!!!

Day 82 Friday, November 29, 2002

Dailiness: holiday; went to see Mom
Time spent: 2 hours
Accountability tip: had two spring rolls for lunch

Day 83 Saturday, November 30, 2002

Dailiness: got up at 4 A.M.; wrote chapter 14
Time spent: 5 hours
Accountability tip: bought healthy foods yesterday for weekend

Day 84 Sunday, December 1, 2002

Dailiness: went to church
Time spent: 6 hours
Accountability tip: healthy lunch—split

CHAPTER 12

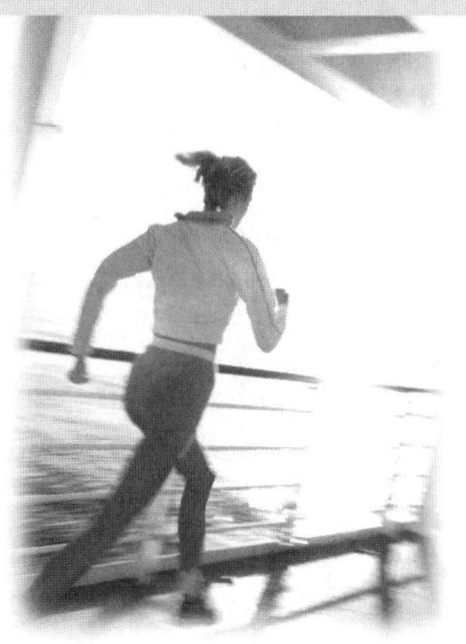

> *There is a time for everything, and a season for every activity under heaven.*
>
> ECCLESIASTES 3:1

LIFE IS DAILY

We never seem to have enough time. No matter how carefully we plan each day, there are always time stealers and time wasters that upset all our best-laid plans. I call this fact of life dailiness. The dailiness of life can keep us from ever becoming the person God planned for us to become. I believe it is the number one reason we get off track in our weight-loss struggle. Paul was speaking of the dailiness of our lives in Romans 7:21: "So I find this law at work: When I want to do good, evil is right there with me."

I am in week 12 of my Triple Dare. I believe I am experiencing almost everything that any of you will experience so that together we can learn how God can help us face the truth of our weight-loss problems. Jesus said in John 8:31-32, "If you hold to my teaching, you are really my disciples. Then you will know the truth, and the truth will set you free." Jesus tells us in these verses that as we obey Him, He will reveal truth to us.

The Dailiness of My Life

Let me explain how the dailiness of my life has played out these past three weeks. I wanted to have this book finished before the busy holiday season got into full swing. To be able to do this, I needed to start writing on November 1. Since I work a full-time job, I would need to find a time to write that didn't interfere with my job. I am not a night person, so it became clear that early mornings would be the time for me to write. To be at my office at 6 A.M. so that I can write for two hours before work begins at 8 A.M. means that I must get up at 4 A.M. in order to leave home at 5 A.M. This means I have no time for my regular exercise routine.

As I started writing, I rationalized that God would help me continue to lose weight, even if I wasn't exercising regularly. What actually happened is that because I wasn't exercising, I also started taking a few liberties with what I ate. First, I ate a few cookies someone left at our house. After one week of writing, I lost a half pound. The next week was much the same: no exercise and a little more playing around with what I ate. At the end of the next week I lost another half pound. By this time we were approaching the 22nd of November, the one-year anniversary of our daughter Shari's death. I did well with my eating on Friday, November 22, and was thrilled that God had scheduled the writing of chapter 10, "Trust God," on that day.

The next day was Saturday, and my daughter Lisa came down to the bay with three of our granddaughters, since we planned to do some Christmas shopping. I needed to go to SAM'S CLUB to buy some large trash bags for Johnny. Everyone wanted to go inside, so we parked the car and all went into the store together.

I had some options available to me. I could have easily gotten the bags, paid for them and waited at the front of the store for the others. Instead of doing that, I wandered through the store until I found them. If you have ever been to SAM'S CLUB on a Saturday, you know that they have free food on every aisle—and my family just happened to be at the free cheesecake aisle when I found them. I had a sliver of cheesecake with them, knowing full well that it was a mistake. Well, what followed was not pretty.

On the next aisle they were serving pumpkin pie and pecan pie, and the woman serving it said, "Take one of each, so you can taste both of them." Of course, I tasted both the pecan pie and the pumpkin pie. I followed the pie with a taste of pizza and then a taste of cranberry bread. By the time we left the store, it was dinnertime but none of us was hungry—for obvious reasons.

We decided to go to a movie that we all had been wanting to see. Because we hadn't eaten dinner, we bought some popcorn and diet sodas to have during the movie. After the movie, we weren't hungry, so we shopped at the mall until midnight—at which time we went to an all-night, fast food restaurant and had breakfast.

Knowing I had to weigh on Monday morning kept me on track all day Sunday; but when I weighed early Monday, I had stayed the same. So here I was: in three weeks I had lost a total of one pound. If I hadn't been writing this book, that would have been the time I got totally off track and started eating everything I wanted. All of us have been there. We start playing around, and before we know it, we're off track and gaining weight again.

I've learned one important truth about weight loss: Anyone can lose weight; gaining weight is the problem. We have all been successful in losing weight time after time. Keeping the weight off is the real challenge.

On Monday of this week, God gave me a real-life example of how daily my life is. I had planned to write Monday through Wednesday and be almost finished with this book by Thanksgiving Day. At noon on Monday, the nurse called from the personal care home where my mom lives and told me that Mom had pulled out her feeding tube. They were calling an ambulance to take her to the hospital, so I said I would meet them there. I arrived at the hospital around 2 P.M. and was there until 10 P.M., when an ambulance came to take her back home. My dinner consisted of a package of cheese crackers from the vending machine. After looking over every item in the machine, this was the healthiest selection—and the six crackers had 10 grams of fat! How many times have we been in a similar situation and we chose the candy bar instead? I have been at the hospital many times with loved ones, and after I purchase that first candy bar, I am destined to get off track.

The Dailiness of Each of Our Lives

What I am saying in this book only applies to those of us who are compulsive overeaters. For compulsive overeaters, there is usually a food that triggers an eating binge. Some people start with a bite of a crunchy food such as chips, while others start with a bite of something sweet. That one bite, many times, is the bite that starts an eating binge. We must know ourselves and what gets us off track if we are to succeed at losing weight and keeping it off.

When we let the interruptions of our daily lives get us off track for days, weeks and months, we get into real trouble: We don't lose weight, and we almost always gain weight.

This is the definition of dailiness: those unexpected things that happen every day that, if you let them, get you off track. In the back of this book you will find journal sheets for your own 16-week Triple Dare. On the top line of each day, you will find the word "dailiness." The purpose of this exercise is to teach each of us that life is daily. Interruptions happen every day. When we let the interruptions of our daily lives get us off track for days, weeks and months, we get into real trouble: We don't lose weight, and we almost always gain weight during these times.

Go back over the last six months of your own life. What are the circumstances that got you off track in losing weight? Was it a job change or a move to a new city? How about an illness? Were there problems with your marriage or children? Are you the primary caregiver for an aging parent? Write your answer here:

The dailiness of life is part of each of our lives. Why don't we accept it as a part of life and get on with becoming the person God wants us to be? God has shown me these last three weeks that He is able: He will help me if I will let Him help me. He will give me a way of escape if I look for it (see 1 Cor. 10:13). Most of my problems in losing weight have to do with me. I am my own worst enemy. In SAM'S CLUB last Saturday, I sacrificed what I want most for what I wanted at the moment. I want to lose all the weight I need to lose in order to bring honor and praise to my Savior, Jesus Christ. Since I wasted three valuable weeks of my 16-week Triple Dare, I now must stay on track every day for the remaining five weeks if I am going to lose the weight. Instead of losing one pound in three weeks, I could have lost five pounds. I now must go through Thanksgiving, Christmas and New Year's without any slipups if I am to finish strong. I pray that the lessons God is teaching me about myself will help each of you who reads this book stay strong.

I don't believe that it is an accident that I am writing this chapter the day before Thanksgiving. Holidays and special occasions are times we can easily get off track. When we think about it, life is full of one special occasion after another. If it isn't a holiday, then it is a birthday celebration, baby shower or wedding reception. Someone brings donuts to the office or pie to Sunday School class. My mom once said, "I had to learn that I couldn't eat up every good thing that comes around, because they just keep on coming."

As you start your own 16-week Triple Dare, watch for your own dailiness. When you do get off track, get right back on and finish strong. Success is in the process. You will succeed if you do not quit.

PRAYER

Dear Lord, the dailiness of my life is a huge problem. Help me look at my own dailiness as the blessing that it is, so I don't grumble and complain. Thank You for my dailiness. I want to lose the weight I need to lose, and I know You'll help me as I believe, trust and obey You. In Jesus' name, amen.

WEEK 13

Weight: 146 **Loss:** 2 pounds

DAY 85 MONDAY, DECEMBER 2, 2002

Dailiness: flew to California; drove to Palm Springs to see Florence
Time spent: 15 hours
Accountability tip: ate healthily

DAY 86 TUESDAY, DECEMBER 3, 2002

Dailiness: Gospel Light sales conference and banquet
Time spent: all day
Accountability tip: ate healthily all day

DAY 87 WEDNESDAY, DECEMBER 4, 2002

Dailiness: gave devotional thoughts at GL sales conference; flew home
Time spent: all day
Accountability tip: ate healthily all day

DAY 88 THURSDAY, DECEMBER 5, 2002

Dailiness: worked all day; went to see Mom
Time spent: 13 hours
Accountability tip: ate healthily

DAY 89 FRIDAY, DECEMBER 6, 2002

Dailiness: stayed after work for birthday party
Time spent: 8 hours
Accountability tip: Chinese food—ate healthily

DAY 90 SATURDAY, DECEMBER 7, 2002

Dailiness: decorated Christmas tree
Time spent: 5 hours
Accountability tip: salad for lunch

DAY 91 SUNDAY, DECEMBER 8, 2002

Dailiness: taught Sunday School
Time spent: 6 hours
Accountability tip: split lunch

Carole's Triple Dare Journal

Week 14

Weight: 145 **Loss:** 1 pound

Day 92 Monday, December 9, 2002

Dailiness: First Place council meeting
Time spent: 5 hours
Accountability tip: ate healthily

Day 93 Tuesday, December 10, 2002

Dailiness: staff Christmas party
Time spent: 2 hours
Accountability tip: ate healthily—no dessert

Day 94 Wednesday, December 11, 2002

Dailiness: planning meetings and haircut
Time spent: 4 hours
Accountability tip:

Day 95 Thursday, December 12, 2002

Dailiness: shopped after work
Time spent: 5 hours
Accountability tip: salad, no dessert—ate at Cheesecake Factory with Cara, Katy and Kay

Day 96 Friday, December 13, 2002

Dailiness: lunch with Jaye
Time spent: 2 hours
Accountability tip: salad and piece of bread

Day 97 Saturday, December 14, 2002

Dailiness: Christmas shopping
Time spent: 5 hours
Accountability tip: ate healthily

Day 98 Sunday, December 15, 2002

Dailiness: church; met Cara and Katy
Time spent: 7 hours
Accountability tip: went to brunch—ate healthily

CHAPTER 13

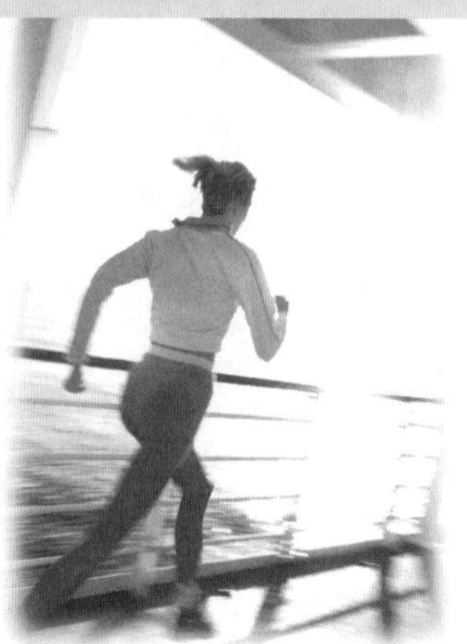

Like a city whose walls are broken down is a man who lacks self-control.

PROVERBS 25:28

PERSONAL ACCOUNTABILITY

If the number one reason we get off track is life's dailiness, then the number two reason is our lack of personal accountability. If we are going to succeed at losing weight and keeping it off, there are major time slots each day that must be adjusted. We must find time each day to spend with God. When we do this, God is able to help us make other good choices throughout the day. Personal accountability means that we

- spend time alone with God each day,
- make wise choices when we select food to eat so that we may have healthy bodies—bodies that bring glory to God,
- exercise regularly to make our bodies strong so that we can serve God for many years to come and
- schedule time for rest and sleep.

If we lack personal accountability in these four areas, we will always struggle to be successful in losing weight and keeping it off.

We have heard it said that integrity is what we do when no one is looking. It is the same with personal accountability. For the last 10 years I have struggled to lose weight; not only that, I gained a few pounds here and there, until I found myself 60 years old, weighing 160 pounds! Since I work with people in the First Place office and lead a First Place class in this same building, I never—let me repeat that, *never*—eat foods that I shouldn't eat in front of these people. My problem has been what I eat on the way home and after I get home and what I eat on weekends.

Personal accountability is what we do when no one is looking. My problem has been what I eat on the way home and after I get home and what I eat on the weekends.

Beverly Henson, who has lost 147 pounds on the First Place program, was in a First Place class for six months and never lost a pound. She was unwilling to exercise because she was so heavy. Beverly had been a competitive swimmer and never had a weight problem until she quit swimming at age 21 and kept eating like a swimmer. She started gaining weight, and she had gained and lost weight so many times that her metabolism was totally out of whack when she joined First Place. Beverly says she was happy to stay the same every week when she weighed at her First Place class meeting. She wasn't losing, but she wasn't gaining either. Beverly says, "I was on maintenance, on the other end." When Beverly finally started walking, she started losing weight every week.

Today, Beverly is the picture of health and has become a certified personal trainer. She swims, kayaks, runs and bikes. She was even named the athlete of the year last year in the Mississippi State Games.

Without personal accountability in our eating and exercise, we will never lose weight and keep it off forever. Some people who join the First Place program start losing weight immediately, and others don't lose weight at all. Many lose two pounds one week and gain it back the next week. The key to success always goes back to personal accountability. We can attend a First Place meeting and receive support and encouragement at the meeting. We can buy healthy foods at the grocery store. We can even purchase fancy exercise equipment so that exercise will be more convenient to our lifestyle. However, without personal accountability, we won't eat the healthy foods we purchased or use the exercise equipment. What we do when we are alone is when we find out how we score in the area of personal accountability.

Writing this book has been an eye-opening experience for me because I have asked God to make me aware of what I do and how easy it is for me to get off track. This is even after I have committed to be honest and up front with each of you who read this book. Old habits are hard to break, and because we are used to giving in to the temptation to eat unhealthy foods, it is also easy not to hold ourselves personally accountable.

God wants us to succeed at losing every pound we need to lose. He also wants us to have a big part in our success. As we obey Him and eat healthy foods, we lose weight. As we exercise daily, we get stronger and feel better.

I have a friend who has suffered from depression for many years; she's been going through a really rough time of depression lately. She was in a First Place class this last session, so she knows what to do. Is she doing it? Of course not! She is eating everything she can get hold of that is sweet or fried. She isn't exercising, because she doesn't feel like it. She isn't spending time alone with God each day, and she isn't sleeping well at night.

Zig Ziglar says, "Feelings follow actions. It is easier to act our way into a new way of feeling than it is to feel our way into a new way of acting."[1]

There is a definite cycle here. Because she is depressed, she lacks the desire to spend time with God. She overeats because she isn't asking God for help. As she overeats, she gains weight. As she gains weight, she is more depressed and has trouble sleeping at night.

Personal accountability breaks the cycle. Get back on track this minute. Make the choice to spend time every day with God. At your next meal, choose healthy food to eat. Put on your walking shoes and head out the front door for a walk. Quit waiting until you feel like it; that will never happen. Start acting like you want to feel, and your feelings will follow.

Time Alone with God

All of us are given the same 24 hours of each day. We each make choices about how we will spend the day. Some days are harder than others, because life is daily and interruptions are part of every day. If we choose to start our day without asking God to help and guide us, we make the worst possible choice we will make all day. Our time with God each

Our time with God each morning must become the single most important item on our personal accountability list.

morning must become the single most important item on our personal accountability list, if we are to experience lasting success in losing weight. We have proven over and over again that we do not have the power to succeed. God has all the power we need, and He will help us if we will only ask Him. Before taking the 16-week Triple Dare to believe, trust and obey God, it would be a great idea to locate a spot in your home where you can meet God each day. Place your Bible, devotional book, prayer journal, pen and whatever tools you will need on the table beside your chosen spot. Having your tools handy makes it easier to have a quality time alone with God.

There are days I wake up late and I'm unable to have my time alone with God in my favorite chair. On those days, I turn off my radio on the drive to work and spend that hour talking to God and listening to God talk to me. Personal accountability means that we find time for the things in our lives that are important to us.

Exercise

Personal accountability means that we find time each day to exercise. For the most part, our society is quite sedentary. We sit in our cars, sit at our desks and sit at home reading the paper or watching TV. Again, we have choices to make all day long about exercise. We can choose to park our car at the far end of the parking lot and walk into the office or store. We can choose to take the stairs instead of the elevator at work. We can choose to give up our paper and TV time to take a walk instead.

There is a price to pay for success. We must always give up something in order to get something better. It has been said, "When we pay the price, the price is mighty nice." Personal accountability means that each day we choose to pay the price. We choose to spend quality time alone with God, and we choose to exercise.

I love to exercise with a friend. My assistant, Pat, and I exercise together most mornings. We meet at our church activities center at 6 A.M. and walk together on treadmills that are side by side. Our physical exercise is what we do to keep our bodies strong, but the most important exercise we do each morning is to practice our Scripture memory verses together. In First Place, we have over 100 memory verses—10 in each Bible study. Pat and I have led First Place together for many years, but it is still necessary for us to regularly practice our verses if they are to be readily available when God needs to bring them out to bless us or someone else each day.

We have our verses on index cards. These cards have two holes punched at the top, with large metal rings holding them together. Each card has the Bible verse on the front and the reference on the back. Pat and I go through the verses taking turns saying each verse while we walk on the treadmill. We have found that it takes about 3 minutes to say 10 verses and we can say all of them in 30 minutes. The time flies by, because our minds are focused on God and not on the walking.

Even though I love exercising with a friend, exercising alone is great, too. I love to walk and pray. I love to walk and sing. Just getting outside for a walk and basking in God's creation is energizing. We can pray for our neighbors as we walk by their homes. We can pray for our own families, for the day ahead and for the choices we will make that day.

Being personally accountable means that each of us must find the time to exercise. We must also find an exercise that we can and will do. Some of us are unable to walk for exercise, but we could ride a stationary bike. Some people reading this book will have 100 pounds to lose or more. If this is the case for you, swimming would be a great way to exercise until you lose enough weight to add other exercises.

A friend of mine has tremendous joint pain because of her excess weight, so she attends a water aerobics class. She says that she has absolutely no pain when she is exercising in the water. Whatever our physical limitations, we can find some way to exercise. If you can barely walk, then barely walk and watch God help you walk a little more every day. Some of you will start by walking down your front walk to the street and back. The next day, ask God to help you walk a little farther. Do whatever you can do, and God will help you do more. God wants to heal our bodies, and He will do it if we will give this problem to Him and ask for His help.

Healthy Eating

Personal accountability in the area of what we choose to eat is vital to our success at losing weight. Thousands of people who are in First Place classes still struggle to lose weight and keep it off because of their food choices. Not once in my life has anyone ever made me eat anything.

I make the choices of what and how much I will eat at least three times each day. Eating is something we all do every day. If we don't eat, we will die. Even though cigarettes, alcohol and drugs are addictive, we can give them up and still live. Food is different; we must eat to live. The problem is that instead of eating to live, many of us have chosen to live to eat. We think constantly about food, always planning the next meal.

By becoming personally accountable to eat healthy foods, we find that our compulsive tendency lessens. It has been my experience that I think compulsively about food because of the type of food I am eating. When I give in to my cravings for something sweet, I constantly think about the next item on my food agenda. By eating healthy foods, we can stop the destructive cycle of bingeing. We won't obsess about eating celery or carrots. When it is time to eat, we will eat healthy foods, if we have committed to become personally accountable in the area of what we eat. Every time we make choices that are good for us, we find that we become stronger. One good choice after another makes one good day. Seven days of wise choices regarding food will spell success when we get on the scales to weigh. Until we learn to be personally accountable in the area of our eating, we will never have the success we desire.

Rest

Rest is another area where we must be personally accountable. We must decide that rest is important and adjust our bedtimes to get the amount of sleep we need. We need a minimum of seven hours each night for maximum productivity.

My life demands that I rise early, so this means I must go to bed early. The other day I was talking to Johnny about a speaking engagement, and I said that I needed to wear something "after five." We both had a good laugh when he said, "This would mean a long nightgown instead of a short one!" I don't go to bed quite that early, but I do start winding down and resting when I get home from work each day.

Because I am at a different season of life from many other people, I have made the choice to eliminate those activities that I can eliminate and spend my leisure time in a state of rest. I try to go by and see my

Mom after work at least three days each week, and many of those days I arrive home physically and emotionally exhausted. Each day when I get home, I change from my work clothes, and Johnny and I spend time on the pier talking and watching the Bowser Boys play. Everything I do after work is calculated to help me wind down after a long day. In doing this, I am assured of a good night's sleep.

There are activities that I used to enjoy doing but that I no longer am able to do, one of which was cross-stitch embroidery. When we were expecting our first grandchild, I did a lot of embroidery. I enjoyed it immensely, but the activity took hours and hours of my time.

I don't want to imply that there is anything wrong with leisure activities. The problem comes when these activities take the place of time spent with God, time spent with our families or time spent exercising. We don't want to spend time doing anything that will keep us from experiencing the success we so desperately want. Remember, we all have the same 24 hours of each day. We must choose how we spend our time.

For me, this time in my own life is a time I need to spend with my precious husband. I don't attend many outside Bible studies, Sunday School class meetings or service clubs. Since Johnny was diagnosed with cancer, we have learned the important lesson of priorities. Most of us think we have forever to do those things that are really important in life, so we spend hours and hours in activities that have very little eternal value. Only when we realize that we could lose something precious—like a loved one or our health—do we value that person or thing enough to spend the time that it deserves. Becoming personally accountable in these four areas will enable us to become the person God can use mightily.

PRAYER

Dear Father, teach me how to be personally accountable. Lead me to someone who has the same need that I have to lose weight and exercise. Teach us how to help each other be personally accountable each day. Thank You in advance for all You are going to do to help me succeed. In Jesus' name, amen.

WEEK 15

Weight: 144 **Loss:** 1 lb.

DAY 99 MONDAY, DECEMBER 16, 2002

Dailiness: on vacation; cleaned house; had company
Time spent: 6 hours
Accountability tip: froze cookies niece brought

DAY 100 TUESDAY, DECEMBER 17, 2002

Dailiness: cleaned house
Time spent: 5 hours
Accountability tip: soup for lunch

DAY 101 WEDNESDAY, DECEMBER 18, 2002

Dailiness: took cat to vet and shopped
Time spent: all day
Accountability tip: got into nuts and candy sent by publisher today

DAY 102 THURSDAY, DECEMBER 19, 2002

Dailiness: went to doctor
Time spent: 2 hours
Accountability tip: still in nuts and candy—get back on track!!!

DAY 103 FRIDAY, DECEMBER 20, 2002

Dailiness: prayed; got back on track
Time spent:
Accountability tip:

DAY 104 SATURDAY, DECEMBER 21, 2002

Dailiness:
Time spent:
Accountability tip: TV program in South Carolina sent 2 pounds of pecans—ack!!!

DAY 105 SUNDAY, DECEMBER 22, 2002

Dailiness:
Time spent:
Accountability tip:

WEEK 16
Weight: 144 **Loss:** stayed the same

DAY 106 MONDAY, DECEMBER 23, 2002
Dailiness:
Time spent:
Accountability tip:

DAY 107 TUESDAY, DECEMBER 24, 2002
Dailiness:
Time spent:
Accountability tip:

DAY 108 WEDNESDAY, DECEMBER 25, 2002
Dailiness:
Time spent:
Accountability tip:

DAY 109 THURSDAY, DECEMBER 26, 2002
Dailiness:
Time spent:
Accountability tip:

DAY 110 FRIDAY, DECEMBER 27, 2002
Dailiness:
Time spent:
Accountability tip:

DAY 111 SATURDAY, DECEMBER 28, 2002
Dailiness:
Time spent:
Accountability tip:

DAY 112 SUNDAY, DECEMBER 29, 2002
Dailiness:
Time spent:
Accountability tip:

MONDAY, DECEMBER 30, 2002
Triple Dare final weight: 144
Total weight loss: 16 pounds

CHAPTER 14

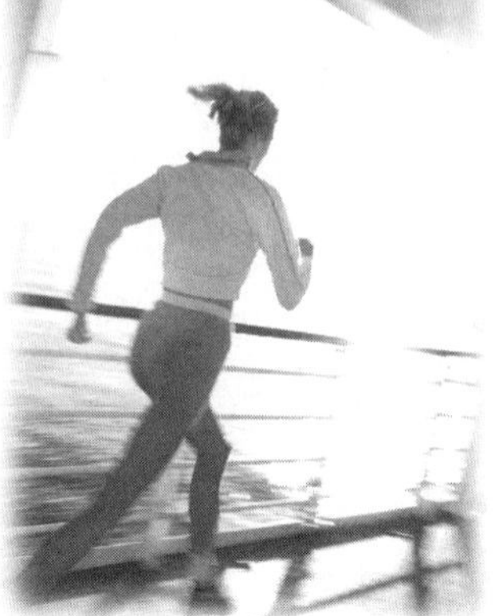

CAROLE'S TESTIMONY

I could not have known all that God would teach me as I sat in my chair the morning of September 9, 2002. As I meditated on John 14:21 and absorbed the truth that Jesus would show Himself to me if I would obey Him, I had no idea that I was in for a 16-week ride of a lifetime. I wish I could say that my journey was a time of complete obedience and that I only chose nutritious, healthy foods to eat. I wish I could say that I exercised every day and did everything right every time I was tempted to get off track.

When God impressed my heart that morning that I needed to be vulnerable and transparent with the people reading this book, you would have thought that I would have been too afraid to get off track—knowing that I would have to write about my failures and defeats right alongside my successes and victories. Quite the opposite happened.

I believe that God allowed every temptation during the entire 16 weeks of the Triple Dare. I also believe that because God knows me so well, He knew I would succumb to temptation and get off track from time to time during the journey. God used these times to teach me things about myself that I won't soon forget. Hopefully, I have learned truths that will help you, the reader, get back on track sooner than you have in your past derailments.

Lessons I Learned by Getting Off Track

I derailed four times during my 16-week Triple Dare. Let me tell you what happened and what I learned about myself.

Vegetable Tempura

I shared in chapter 1 my first derailment with the vegetable tempura. Here's what I learned from the experience:

I don't make good choices when I'm tired.

When I am tired, my defenses are down and I don't care whether I make the best choices. First Corinthians 10:13 says that God will always provide a way of escape so that we are able to stand up under temptation. During these times, I won't get off track if I choose to take God's way of escape. Here are three things I learned from my tempura derailment that I can do the next time I'm tempted when I'm tired:

1. Tell God I'm tired and ask for His strength.
2. Decide what I will eat before going inside the restaurant.
3. Excuse myself and go into the rest room, asking someone to order for me, so I am not tempted to change my mind.

Cookie Escapade

Weeks 9 and 10 were two weeks when I dabbled with a box of cookies left at my house. You won't see the cookies on my journal entries—except at the end of week 10. Inside the box were four cellophane-wrapped bags, each containing two cookies. These were not ordinary cookies; they were the gourmet variety. After eating the first two cookies one night when I was tired, I found myself drawn to the cookies every few days. Each time, I opened the cellophane wrapper and ate two cookies. I did this until the box was empty. I never told Johnny or Kay, who was my houseguest at the time, what I was doing, and I never asked for help. I felt compelled to eat those cookies until every last one was gone. Notice on weeks 10 and 11 of my journal that I lost a half pound each week. On week 12, I stayed the same.

From my cookie escapade I learned:

I get off track when I eat in secret.

When I am secretive about what I eat, I am only fooling myself. I didn't write in my journal what I was doing because I thought no one would know. After all, it was only eight cookies! Here are five more things I learned from my cookie derailment:

1. "What I eat in secret is there for the entire world to see what a fool I am" (a phrase I heard said many years ago at a weight-loss group).
2. Secret eating is the most lethal kind of derailment. I can be good when someone is watching, but I can get off track fast when I eat in secret.
3. My way of escape was to tell Johnny or Kay what I was doing. They would have gotten rid of the cookies for me.
4. Don't open the first cellophane wrapper of anything that you know is delicious. Leave the food in the wrapper!
5. My mind is the battlefield that the enemy used in the cookie derailment. I knew that those cookies were still available. Once I started thinking about them, eating them wasn't far behind.

Christmas Foods That Came in the Mail

I was on vacation from December 16 until January 6. Not only would three weeks at home, during the holidays, have been reason enough to get off track, but also the weather was cold, gray and dreary, and my mom was dying in a personal care home.

On December 18, a big box arrived from our publisher. I excitedly opened the box and found a beautiful basket wrapped in cellophane. Inside the basket were all the new books that had been released the previous three months. Along with the books were two items that not only had the potential to cause a derailment, but they could have caused a train wreck! In my publisher's defense, they use an outside company to send the current books to their authors every quarter, and the company does a gorgeous job of packaging them. The books are always wrapped individually, with beautiful papers and bows. I'm sure that since it was Christmas, the company decided to put in a couple of treats as a special Christmas gift.

Well, inside the basket was an eight-ounce box of chocolates and a one-pound can of salted mixed nuts. The chocolates and the nuts were wrapped in cellophane and would have been a welcome treat at Mom's personal care home, had I made the choice to take them there when I went to visit her. Did I do this? Not on your life! You see, when I was a child, one of my grandmothers lived in California. I only saw her once a year, so she kept in touch by sending me chocolates. At Easter, a box would arrive with eight beautiful, chocolate Easter eggs. As a child, I didn't have a problem with sweets, but I remember the white, rectangular box with Easter grass and the beautifully decorated eggs. Seeing that box of chocolates brought memories of my grandmother that were sweet and full of nostalgia. I hope you see where I'm going here.

Let me share what I learned after getting derailed on chocolates and nuts:

> My mind is filled with warm memories related to food.

Here are three other things I learned from this chocolate and nut derailment:

1. Getting off track is easy when memories are tied to unhealthy foods.

2. If I stop to thank God for the sweet memories and ask for His strength, He will help me break the connection between the memory and the food.
3. I derive comfort from soft and creamy foods. If I have candy around during a bleak, sad time, I am setting myself up for a derailment—actually, candy is hard for me to resist anytime.

After two days of eating the chocolates and nuts, I asked God for help to get back on track. I went by our office on December 21, and Nancy and Stephanie, two of my coworkers, said that a package had come for me. They had checked out the contents, and Nancy said, "I don't know if you should take this home. You might get off track." I assured Nancy that I would be fine, and I left the office with the box. When I arrived home, I opened the box to find that a TV station had sent me two pounds of pecans! There were three different bags, containing three varieties. One bag contained orange-flavored pecans, another cinnamon flavored and the third bag plain, salted pecans. The company uses sugar to make the flavorings stick to the pecans—you can imagine how good they tasted.

In hindsight, I see the enemy's thumbprints all over this gift of pecans. The enemy's primary goal in the life of a Christian is to kill, rob and destroy. He was working overtime the last few weeks of my Triple Dare to see that I would have a weak finish. The funny thing about this is that I kept encouraging the other Triple Dare participants to finish strong!

Like the chocolates and mixed nuts, the pecans were a thoughtful gift, and the sender was certainly not the enemy. I disagree when people blame the devil every time they get off track, so sometimes I mistakenly ignore the truth that he uses things to try to get me to fail.

The enemy can never make us get off track without our permission. God tells us in His Word that Satan leads the whole world astray and that he accuses us before God day and night (see Rev. 12:9-10). God has the power to help us resist. We always have the ability to make a wise, rather than a foolish, choice.

Why, then, do I think that the enemy was involved? First, I have never received a gift after an appearance on any TV station—and I have appeared on quite a few stations. Second, I was not even scheduled to be on this particular TV station's show until June, and this was December! To say that I was flattered and appreciative is an understatement. I was absolutely floored that the station was so thoughtful. See how we can be set up?

God was faithful and used the pecans to teach me still more truths. Here are two I learned about our enemy, the devil:

He knows our weakness and he wants us to fail.

What can we do to foil the attack?

1. Run to God when we suspect that the enemy is trying to get us off track.
2. Ask God for help and for the wisdom to stop. Better still, ask God for help before we start! The only thing I tried was begging three of my granddaughters to finish the pecans when they came to visit.
3. Take the way of escape. My way of escape was to put a Christmas bow on each of the bags and to give a bag each to three of our neighbors as a thoughtful Christmas gift.
4. Remember: *Don't open the cellophane!*
5. Keep filling out the accountability journal. Once I stopped filling out my journal (during the fifteenth week), my accountability went out the window.

My Prayer for You

I hope these sad stories don't leave you with the impression that the entire Triple Dare was a defeat. It was a glorious time of victory *when* I asked God for help. The first eight weeks were wonderful. As I was obedient, God helped me stay on track. But when I let down my guard and ate the first nibble of the foods that God and I had decided were off-limits for me during those 16 weeks, I was setting myself up for a derailment. At the end of the 16 weeks, I had lost 16 pounds.

My prayer for each of you as you read this book is that God will use my mistakes to teach you some valuable lessons about yourself. I daresay, most of you will see yourself in my foolishness. Maybe you will even see that none of us is really very different from the other.

The primary thing we must all learn if we are to have permanent victory in the area of weight loss is that if we will obey our heavenly Father, He will be true to His Word and show Himself to us (see John 14:21).

APPENDIX A

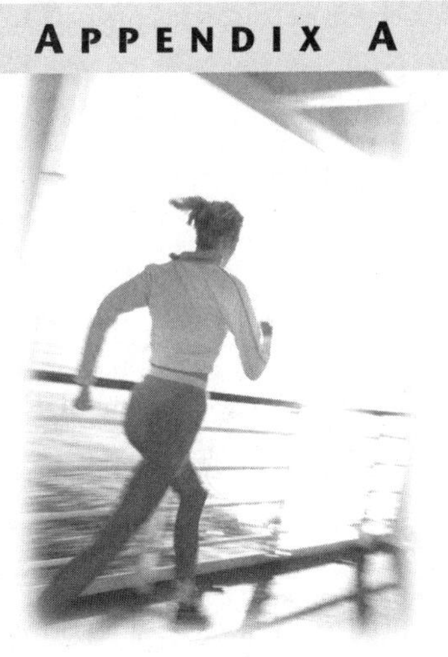

THE TRIPLE DARE PLAN

ACCOUNTABILITY AND SUPPORT

Accountability is the key to success in the Triple Dare. Ideally, it would be great to find a friend or relative willing to take the Triple Dare with you for 16 weeks. In doing this, you could exchange *commitment forms* and hold each other accountable each week. You may photocopy the commitment form, located on page 121, for this purpose. You may want to increase the image to 130 percent to fit a standard sheet of paper.

If it is not possible to do the Triple Dare with someone else, fill out the commitment form and tell God about your commitment, asking Him to help you be accountable to Him each week.

In addition, *First Place* has *groups* all over the world. Go to our website, www.firstplace.org, and type in your zip code to find a group to join. We also have online groups for those who are unable to attend a class.

A Triple Dare *bulletin board* is available on our website so that you can give and receive encouragement on your 16-week journey. To get to the Triple Dare bulletin board, get on the Internet and type in www.firstplace.org/tripledare.

User ID: tripledare
Password: Believe

The First Place *e-newsletter* is another means of encouragement for you. Sign up on the First Place website.

The Plan

The 16-week Triple Dare is not a complicated plan, and your making wise personal choices is the key to your success. We are going to believe God, trust God and obey God for 16 weeks. If we are to succeed, there are six major things we must do.

Time Alone with God

Set aside a time and place each day to spend time alone with God. If the dailiness of life gets in the way, carve out another time slot before you go to bed. Time with God must be a priority if we are to succeed.

Healthy Eating

The eating plan is extremely simple. Eat healthy foods such as fruits and vegetables. We didn't get fat from eating too many fruits and vegetables, so eat all you want–in moderation. Eat fruits and vegetables as close to their natural state as possible. Use low-calorie salad dressings.

Eat complex carbohydrates, such as whole-grain bread, pasta, rice and potatoes. You may eat seven to eight servings of these each day. A serving is one slice of bread or half a cup.

Consume only low-fat meats and dairy products. Eat five to six ounces of lean meat or low-fat cheese each day. Consume two to three eight-ounce servings of nonfat or low-fat milk or yogurt. Season your food with spices, not with butter or bacon. Use moderation in the amounts of meats and dairy you eat.

Do not eat high-calorie desserts or chips. Do not eat fried foods. Do not eat creamy salads. If you do eat these foods during the Triple Dare, immediately get back on track before you derail.

Drink eight glasses of water each day. Do not drink high-calorie drinks of any kind.

Exercise

Do not go longer than 48 hours without some kind of exercise. If you can barely walk, then barely walk. God will reward your efforts. Find an exercise you enjoy and do it. If you have 100 pounds to lose or more, find a place to swim.

Exercise five days a week. Most of us work or go to school five days a week, so a five-day exercise schedule can become a part of our five-day workweek. Do not debate whether or not you will exercise. Make an appointment to exercise at least five days each week, and keep the appointment. Remember, showing up is 80 percent of life. Show up, start, and you will finish. Our goal is to work up to being able to walk 12 to 15 miles each week.

Rest

Adjust your schedule so that you can get seven to eight hours of sleep each night. Proper rest will allow you to keep the other priorities of having a quiet time, eating properly and exercising each day. Learn to rest and play during this 16-week Triple Dare. Rest and play are miracle workers for our emotional health because they help us deal with the stressors of our daily life.

Journal

A one-week, blank journal is included on page 122 for you to photocopy. Make a copy for each of the 16 weeks of the Triple Dare, and take a few minutes each day to fill it in. Jot down your own dailiness and how long you spent doing whatever you hadn't planned to do. Dailiness might also be something positive that is particularly rewarding, like a great quiet time. Those quality times with God result in time saved instead of time spent. Record in your journal one area each day where you held yourself personally accountable. It might be a good choice in the food you ate or a small addition to your daily exercise routine.

Weekly Weigh-In

Weigh yourself on the same day and at the same time each week. Better still, ask someone else to weigh you. This adds more personal accountability. Record your weight each week. If your weight stays the same or increases one week, work harder the next week. Get right back on track.

It is *important to remember* that physiologically it is impossible to lose more than two pounds of fat each week. If after three weeks you are losing more than two pounds per week, you are losing lean body mass (the mechanism that gives your body energy and strength). Increase your food intake until you are losing only one and one-half to two pounds each week.

After the Triple Dare Ends

If you need to lose more weight than you can lose in 16 weeks, you'll want to keep doing the 16-week Triple Dare until you reach your weight goal. By the time you reach your goal, you will have established habits that will help you keep the weight off forever. You'll also have a closer walk with God than you'd ever dreamed possible.

Congratulations. You have chosen to undertake the most exciting adventure of your life. I'm praying for your success.

Prayer

Dear Father, You know how many times I have failed in the past. I desperately want this to be the last time I lose weight. Help me learn Your ways as I believe, trust and obey You. Show me Your plan for my life. In Jesus' name, amen.

TRIPLE DARE COMMITMENT

Name ____

Mailing Address ____________________________________

City ________________________ State ______ Zip ____________

Phone–Daytime _________________ Evening __________________

E-Mail Address _________________________

Beginning Date ________________

Beginning Weight ______________

Measurements at the Largest Point:

Ankle:

Calf:

Knee:

Thigh:

Hips:

Waist:

Bust:

Wrist:

Upper Arm:

I, ____________________________________ (name), have accepted the Triple Dare and will faithfully keep my commitment to believe, trust and obey God for the next 16 weeks, beginning today, ______________(date).

I commit to spending some time each day alone with God.
I commit to eating healthy foods and to exercising for the next 16 weeks.
I commit to getting enough rest and sleep each day.
I commit to getting back on track immediately, whenever I am tempted to quit.

____

(signature)

TRIPLE DARE JOURNAL

Week ___
Weight _____ Loss _____ Gain _____

Day ___ **Date** ____________________
Dailiness:
Time spent:
Accountability tip:

Day ___ **Date** ____________________
Dailiness:
Time spent:
Accountability tip:

Day ___ **Date** ____________________
Dailiness:
Time spent:
Accountability tip:

Day ___ **Date** ____________________
Dailiness:
Time spent:
Accountability tip:

Day ___ **Date** ____________________
Dailiness:
Time spent:
Accountability tip:

Day ___ **Date** ____________________
Dailiness:
Time spent:
Accountability tip:

Day ___ **Date** ____________________
Dailiness:
Time spent:
Accountability tip:

APPENDIX B

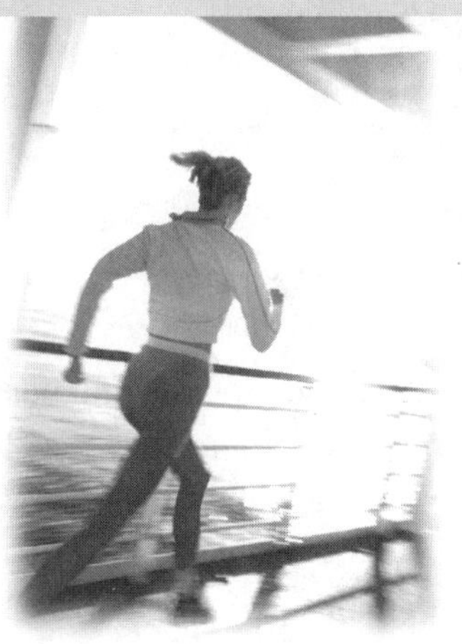

TEN TRIPLE DARE TESTIMONIES

First Place received testimonies from many wonderful people who took the Triple Dare. Unfortunately, we were not able to include all of their testimonies in this book, but we would still like to honor them:

Bessie Lewis from Enterprise, Louisiana, lost 7 pounds.
Betty McPhail from Starkville, Mississippi, lost 10 pounds.
Danielle King from Loveland, Ohio, lost 16¼ pounds.
Ella Lahm from Saint Clair, Missouri, lost 19 pounds.
Kathy Runion from Greer, South Carolina, was not able to exercise because of Lyme disease.
Martha Norsworthy from Murray, Kentucky, lost 11¾ pounds.

Shelley Wilburn from West Frankfort, Illinois, lost 10 pounds.
Sherry Davis from Choctaw, Oklahoma, lost 7 pounds.

ALLIE

SAN ANTONIO, TEXAS

I went to Fitness Week with the expectation and desire that the Lord would give me a great time of weight loss. Imagine my surprise when He did so much more! I had been through several years of chronic depression, a most unhappy marriage and physical problems—uterine and cervical cancer, diabetes and other associated problems of obesity. Today, after successfully completing the Triple Dare, I rejoice that I am a new person in the Lord. Let me tell you about it.

I arrived at Round Top thinking and feeling, *Woe is me.* I was angry at myself for letting myself become a physical wreck—more than 100 pounds over a healthy weight. I had been in the tomb of depression for at least 10½ years of my 11-year marriage, feeling that it was a terrible mistake on both of our parts to give up a friendship of 25 years for a miserable relationship that hadn't been satisfying to either one of us. Spiritually, I had only been attending church again for about nine months after a 20-year hiatus that I took because I had the audacity to stay mad at God for something that happened in the early '80s. Mentally, I knew that if something didn't change soon, the small thread of hope that I had left—to experience joy and meaning in my life—would break and perhaps lead to further disaster.

Carole's challenge to believe, trust and obey was just what I needed to help me focus on a solution to, instead of simply focusing on, all my problems. After the meeting the second night, I went back to my room, got on my knees and sobbed to our almighty heavenly Father, "I give up! I surrender this anger, these disappointments, these bad choices, this lack of belief, trust and obedience to Your will and leave it all at Your feet. Please forgive me for not giving You first place in my life. From this day forward I want You to grow me and mold me as You see fit for Your service." As the week progressed and I listened to the speakers, participated in the worship and fellowship, did the Bible studies and exercised, a peace and joy came over me that is beyond ordinary explanation.

I lost 7¼ pounds that week and 16 pounds total during the Triple Dare. Every day I continue to meet my heavenly Father in prayer and Bible study. I look better, feel better, think better and worship in true thankfulness that God can do for us what we cannot do for ourselves—if we ask and then let Him help us to believe, trust and obey Him.

Cheri Lasiter

Fulshear, Texas

I have cerebral palsy and I walk with the aid of canes. I've had a weight problem all my life, and every time I tried to lose weight and keep it off, I didn't succeed.

By the year 2000, my life had become very complicated. I was unemployed and unable to find something I could do. While my physical health was generally good, I became plagued with increasing stiffness and arthritis in my feet. In fact, it became harder for me to get around at all because it was too hard to exercise. I had always tried to be independent, so my increasing lack of mobility was very discouraging.

My life became out of control and full of despair. Withdrawing from activities and people, I often sat alone in my apartment with the shades down and curtains closed. The darkness of the room began to represent the darkness invading my soul. As I became more lonely and out of control, food became a way of escape. I consumed whole cakes in one or two days. I was so tired physically, emotionally and spiritually that if I had ever been prone to suicidal tendencies, this would have been the time.

Sunday afternoon, February 20, 2001, I felt discouraged with everything. Becoming fearful of how my life was heading, I cried out to the Lord for help. I told Him I was very lonely and asked Him to bless me with one new friend. The next morning I had a divine wake-up call. While listening to my radio, I heard the announcer introduce a woman named Nancy Taylor, who was interviewed about a First Place anniversary. My mind went back to the time I had attended First Place with a friend. Suddenly, the First Place logo with the words "physical," "mental," "emotional" and "physical" popped in my mind. I thought I needed help in all those areas, so I wrote down Nancy's telephone number.

I began my First Place experience April 3, 2001, arriving at First Baptist Church absolutely scared to death. When I went into that first meeting, there was such a feeling of love, warmth and genuine compassion that it was like the Lord Himself was there hugging me. I felt overwhelmed hearing about all of the First Place commitments, so I concentrated first on the attendance commitment—the other commitments eventually fell into place.

My success has been absolutely supernatural! Since April 2001, I have missed only one meeting, and it isn't as much of a struggle to walk and stand on my feet now. The Lord has also taken away many of my fears, as He has been transforming me through His love. He has filled my heart with a new confidence, a new boldness and a new love for Him on this First Place journey.

Carole Lewis presented the Triple Dare at our First Place halftime celebration last year. I was so afraid of failing—because I knew the holidays were upon us—that I didn't commit right away. Though I was very close to my goal weight (the Lord has given me much success), I knew in my heart that I was not where I wanted to be. I had struggled with the last few pounds and felt a real sense of need for this kind of challenge. I also wanted to be a part of what Carole was doing, because I knew the Lord would also be there.

A few more days passed, and the deadline was close, so I decided that I would commit to the challenge and just do the best I could. I remember trying to be so perfect during the Thanksgiving holidays, only to lose sight of making wise choices. Lunches with friends were loaded with starchy vegetables and sweets, and at one point I was offered candy corn and ate three handfuls. I came back from Thanksgiving with a five-pound gain.

Christmas was stressful for me, so I asked God to keep me motivated. He was faithful to bring to mind Carole's saying that life is a series of beginning agains. She said that success is just being able to begin again more quickly. My life has been a series of beginning agains. I had to begin again as I learned to walk and strengthen my muscles. I would not be walking today if I had not gotten up after each fall or surgery and

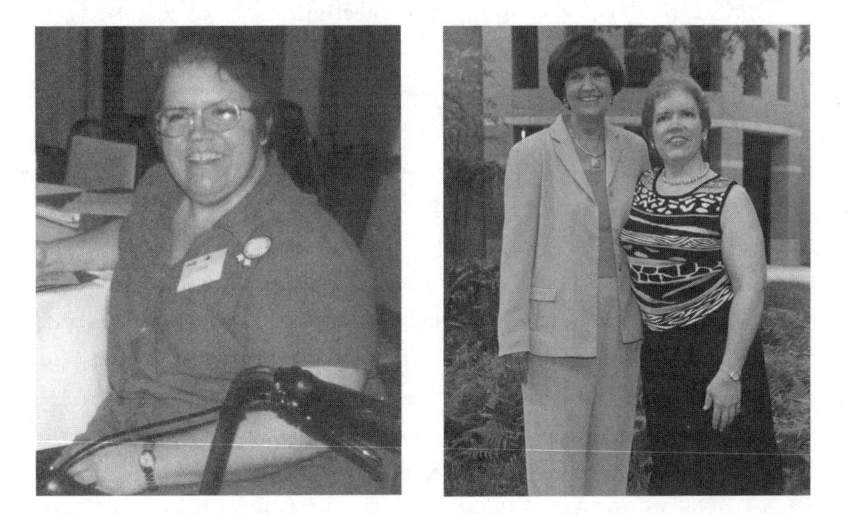

begun again. Remembering this was a great encouragement. I immediately got back on track and lost weight during the Christmas holidays.

I believe I would not have been able to begin again had I not committed to this challenge. On February 4, 2003, I weighed in at my First Place meeting and was one pound under my goal. I have lost a total of 77 pounds.

Janet Kirkhart

Mount Orab, Ohio

When I heard Carole present the Triple Dare, I felt that God had planned it just for me. As a First Place leader for nine years, I had lost 50 pounds; and then, during a long season of loss in my life, I gained most of it back. I knew that even though God had radically changed my life spiritually, mentally and emotionally, it was time to work on the physical.

As I began the Triple Dare, I was able to keep the commitments and consistently lose weight because I started to weigh, measure my exchanges, exercise and cook meals at home using the First Place recipes. Everything was going great until my husband, Kenny, took an early layoff from work because of spurs on his feet and arthritis in his knees. My whole routine was thrown off, so I neglected consistent exercise (another lie from Satan that I used as an excuse). I gained back three pounds, but I was determined not to give up. I made a serious commitment and told God that this time had to be different.

As I was praying before getting ready for church on November 10, my husband called me to come quickly. We saw a perfect rainbow in the field behind our house; every color was brilliant and a complete arch—it was the most beautiful rainbow I had ever seen. I commented to Kenny, "That is God's promise to us." As I returned to my quiet time, God told me that this was a sign of His promise to me that when I fail and fall, He will be there; when I obey, get up and immediately get back on track, He will give me victory. I promised to do this for 16 weeks, and He promised to be there every step of the way. I knew I could not and would not quit.

I have struggled at times since that day, gaining a pound or two and then losing it. During Thanksgiving and Christmas, I used First Place dessert recipes and did not eat high-fat food, although my portion sizes were too large. Unable to attend water aerobic classes at the YMCA because of a three-week break in classes, I did not get enough exercise and I gained four pounds. Again, God was faithful, and I got back on track more quickly than before. I lost the four pounds and continued to lose slowly.

I have learned so much about myself during First Place—even more during the Triple Dare. During my quiet times, I asked God and myself, *What makes this different?* I believe it is the prayer, support and accountability. I also find it helps to keep reminders constantly in front of me. I keep the "Believe" pillow that Carole gave each of us at Round Top Fitness Week on my desk, so I can see it when I study or talk on the phone. I wear my First Place "Believe, Trust and Obey" bracelet every day. The song "I Gotta Believe" by Yolanda Adams has become my Triple Dare theme song, because its lyrics are perfect for this challenge. These reminders keep me focused on my goal and on the victory at the finish line.

My goal was to lose 20 pounds, which I could have easily reached had I been more faithful and consistent; however, I am praising God for what He has done. I lost 17½ pounds during the Triple Dare, making a total of 41 pounds lost since January 2002. I am now in a regular size and do not have to shop in the plus-size sections. What a milestone and victory!

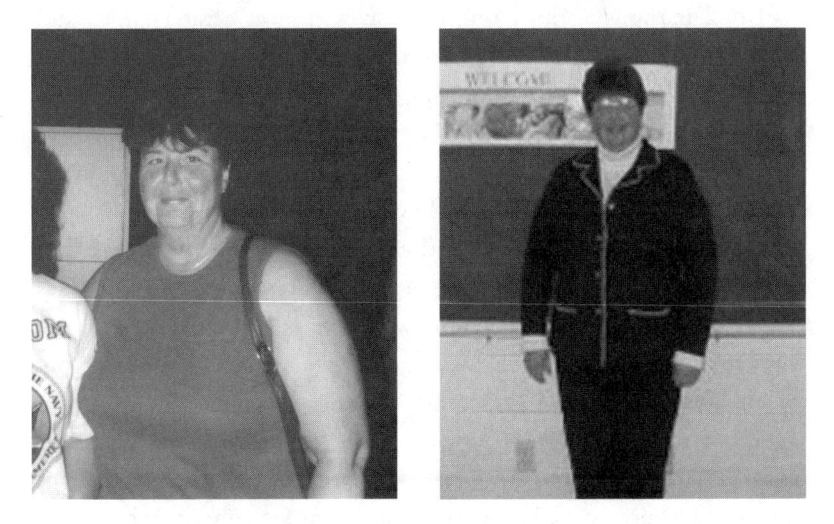

I am so thankful to Carole and all of the staff at First Place for their prayers and encouragement. First Place is like a family to me. Most of all, I am thankful and praising God for what He is doing in my life to change me from the inside out. I can hardly wait to begin Triple Dare II.

Karey Lookadoo

Hot Springs, Arkansas

I joined First Place in July 2002, and I'd lost 27 pounds before I accepted the Triple Dare in September 2002. I lost those pounds in just one session, so when I was presented with the challenge to believe, trust and obey, I thought it would be easy—I couldn't have been more wrong.

Through the Triple Dare, the Lord blessed me by helping me lose 10 pounds, bringing my total loss to 37 pounds. Only by God's grace and mercy did I lose those 10 pounds. The word "challenge" does not begin to describe my 16-week journey. I fell several times and as a result gained pounds during those times. There were times that I got right back on track and other times that it took me a little longer, but I always started again.

I had many victories along the way. One was after Halloween. I came home one day, having a hard time and really craving chocolate. As I walked in, I saw a shopping bag full of my favorite chocolate candies on top of the refrigerator. My husband, who is not usually a chocolate kind of person, had been to the store and loaded up on the sale candy. I couldn't believe it. I told him he was of the devil—lovingly, of course—and told him to get that stuff out of the house, which he quickly did. I never knew where he hid his stash and I never asked. Many times I would see the empty wrappers in the trash for the next few weeks, but the Lord gave me strength over my desire to search out the chocolate treasure.

The hardest times for me were after the Thanksgiving and Christmas holidays. There were so many goodies left over, and I hated to see them go to waste—I love sweets a lot! So with all the guests gone and these wonderful desserts left behind, I knew I had to do something. I asked my husband to be my conscience by asking me if I really needed a second helping of food or something sweet when he saw that I had it. Reluctantly, he did as I asked, and, I have to tell you, many times I was not happy about it. One evening while my husband was in the shower, I went to the kitchen and ate some things I didn't need—but wanted. I knew he would have stopped me if he had seen me eating them. The next morning I awoke with this verse in my head: "You know my folly, O God; my guilt is not hidden from you" (Ps. 69:5).

It took me awhile, but did I ever get the message. I felt so guilty and asked my gracious, heavenly Father to forgive me. I got up and got back on track; and I don't sneak anymore, because I know that even if no one else sees, God does.

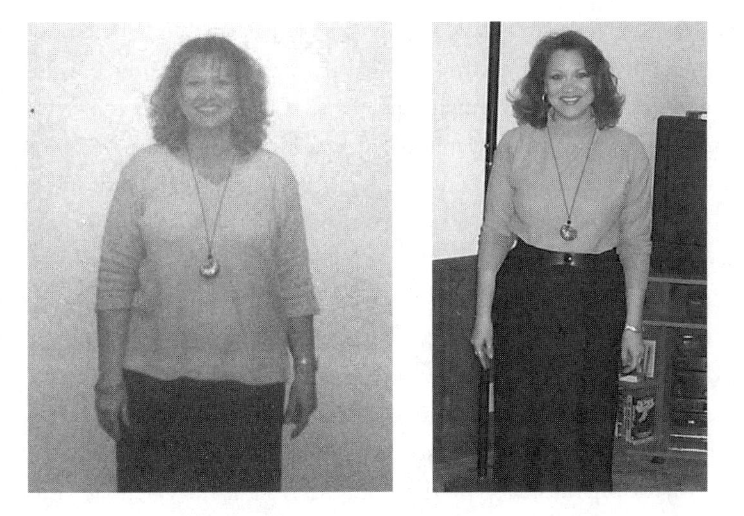

I still struggle with my flesh, and God is gracious to allow me to start again and again. He will never forsake me in this battle and will always be by my side to pick me up when I fall.

KATHY HICKEY

CLARKSVILLE, ARKANSAS

Although I've been in First Place for over six years, life threw me a curve when my only grandchild, Madeline, was born with a rare disease. For the three years that we fought to keep her alive, food often became my stress reliever. After she died, it often became my comforter.

As God healed my grief, I was able to get back on track, and after two sessions, I had lost 20 pounds. Then I got stuck for the next two and didn't lose any! Knowing what it would take, God led me to Fitness Week, where I took the Triple Dare.

I was alarmed when I realized that my 16-week commitment included the holidays! Although *every year* I vowed that *this year* would be different, my first indulgence always triggered a binge that lasted from Thanksgiving until New Year's Day! My records show that I gained an average of 10½ pounds in each of the seven previous holiday seasons.

However, the Bible says that *nothing* is impossible with God—even falling *seven times* and getting up again! The morning after Carole gave us the challenge, I was praying as always for God to set me free from bondage to compulsive overeating, when He spoke to my heart, telling me never to ask that again, because *it was done!* And He gave me a new message: "Say to the captives, 'Come out,' and to those in darkness, 'Be free!'" (Isa.49:9).

It seemed like a miracle that I didn't struggle much with food during the holidays. It wasn't easy to pass on my former binge foods, but I loved being *free!* It felt like a surreal dream to get on the scales and watch the numbers go down instead of up! I even lost weight during the weeks of Thanksgiving, Christmas and an 1,800-mile road trip—what I call my Triple Miracles! By the time I looked at the calendar and realized the Triple Dare was over, I had lost 15 pounds!

Later, while I talked to some people in a Christian 12-step program about the "strange miracle" God had done, a man smiled and said, "I bet if you go back and look through your journals, you'll see lesson after lesson that God has taught you, step after step that you've taken." He said that each lesson and each step were like God's peeling off another layer of an onion. I realized that it was my six years in First Place that had brought me to that moment of freedom, not just some special "zap from God."

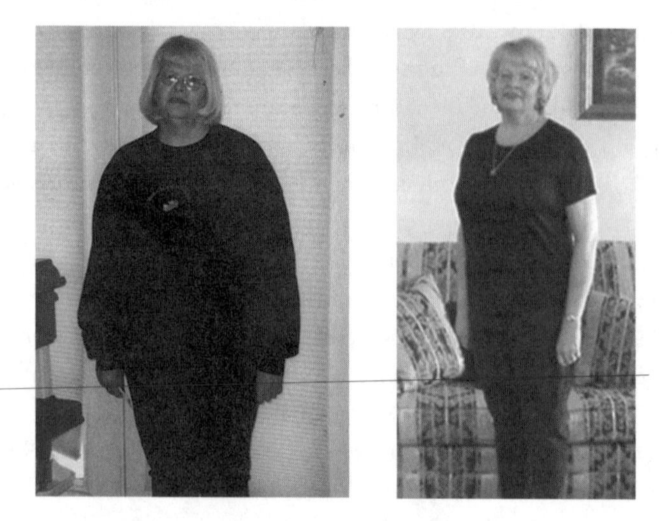

Through my experience with First Place, I have learned not to give up. My struggle to be free from food addiction has not been immediate, nor has it been easy, but God is setting me free!

Kay Smith

Roscoe, Texas

I heard about the Triple Dare for the first time at Carole's house in Houston on the way to Hattiesburg, Mississippi, for the First Place conference. Each time Carole began to tell me about this plan, she would get so excited, but I did not understand her excitement—I was much like the witnesses at Pentecost, who did not understand the effect the Holy Spirit can have on our lives. My recurring thought was, *Why do we need the Triple Dare if we are already in First Place?* But as I listened to Carole's testimony at the conference and pondered on believing God, trusting God and obeying God, I realized that I could use the challenge. I was believing and trusting God, but I knew I was not doing my best to obey God.

As a member of First Place, I lost 90 pounds over four years; however, over the past 15 years I gained back more than 30. I reasoned that the 30-pound weight gain was not a big deal because 60 pounds was still a good loss, and I knew that the loss could not compare to the benefits of spiritual growth and emotional healing that I reap each day of my First Place journey. During those years, I always believed that First Place works as a weight-loss program, and I always led a group. If I gained a pound or two, I was very lenient on myself, thinking, *With what you are going through, it could have been five.* Many weeks I could have made better food choices, or I only exercised one or two days. I never thought of myself as off track; rather, I thought of myself as not as obedient as I could be. Actually, not gaining all the weight back has been a victory for me in First Place, because I had lost weight in other programs but gained it back in less time than it took to lose it. My greatest enemy was telling myself, *I will do better tomorrow.* I had to be honest: I was not doing my best. I began to like this idea of a special challenge.

I began to feel the excitement about this challenge that I had seen in Carole, while flying to Houston to attend the First Place Fitness Week. While I was studying the memory verses we would learn at Fitness Week, God spoke a special word to me as I read Deuteronomy 30. In my Bible, the chapter's heading says "Restoration dependent on repentance." The verses convicted me of my disobedience, and I prayed a prayer of confession, asking God to help me live verse 6 each day. As I read verse 19, "This day I call heaven and earth as witnesses against you that I have set before you life and death, blessings and curses. Now, choose life, so that you and your children may live," the word "now" stood out to me. It came, not in a harsh tone, but in a loving voice from the Father. The heading above these verses says, "The crucial choice before them." I have always believed in the program, but many times I had not chosen to be faithful *now.* I had a special word from God, and I chose to act *now.*

During my 16-week Triple Dare, I lost 16 pounds. I believe it was no accident that we were asked to do it through the Thanksgiving and Christmas holidays. We celebrated Thanksgiving at our home with Joe's family. His mom is famous for her pies and cakes, and I was able to avoid these delicious desserts by preparing a huge fruit salad. Each time I was tempted, I ate a bowl of fruit salad with a little whipped topping, so I did not feel deprived. The fruit salad was so good that I kept some prepared for Joe and me throughout the holidays.

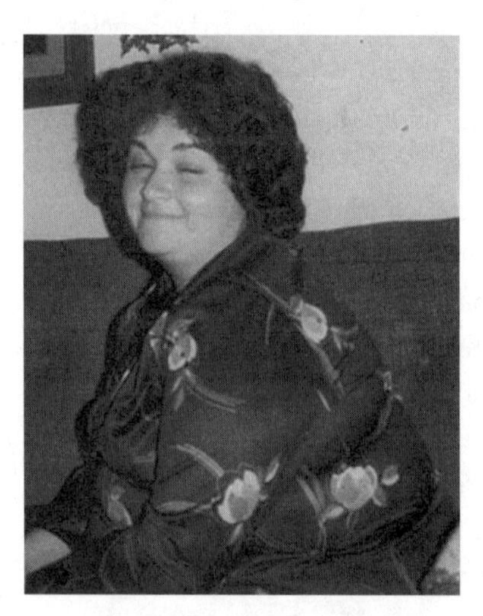

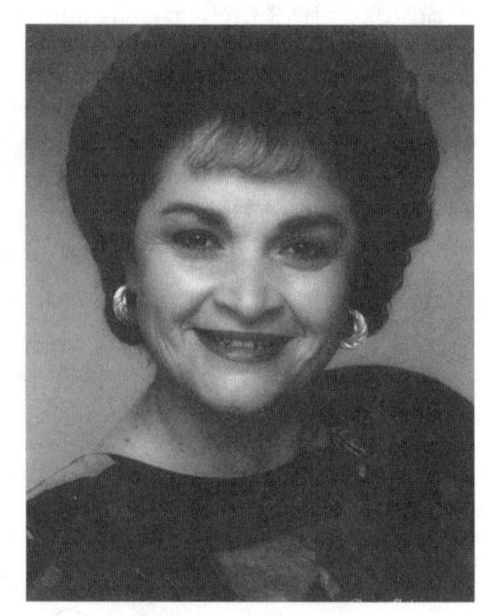

In times past, I've baked as many as 50-dozen cookies and filled boxes for friends and family. We now share Joe's special salsa instead of cookies. I do make a batch of Joe's favorite and a batch of sugar cookies for the grandkids to decorate when they arrive for Christmas, but they're not a temptation because I don't like Joe's favorite, and if you could see the four grandkids up on the cabinet making those cookies, you wouldn't be tempted to eat them either.

I completed my first Triple Dare, and I'm thankful for this special challenge to do what I already know to do.

Lavahn Stillwell

Shreveport, Louisiana

Out of all the nine First Place commitments, exercise has been very hard for me. My stubborn spirit never could get me truly motivated; my "wanna" button said, "No thanks!" But God and I started out the 2002 fall session differently. I was more pliable, more open, as God and I exercised together; but I still seemed to have just an "I've gotta do this!" type attitude.

Then I went to the Mississippi conference and something happened—a real miracle occurred inside me! Was it because of the ongoing progress already at work in my life? Was it the things shared by each of the Houston First Place leaders at the conference? Was it Dr. Couey's challenge to get in there and make exercise work for *me?* I believe all of these things had a part in the miracle. And though I don't know all that went on inside me that weekend, I do know that the conference and Carole's Triple Dare made many differences in my heart and life, and I'll never be the same.

The biggest miracle is the new way I feel about exercise. Now for me, it's just like eating breakfast: I do it because I *want to* do it—for Him! I don't have to talk myself into it; I am compelled to do it from the inside. During many weeks, I'll exercise more within one day than I'd ever thought possible. Exercise is nourishment, just like food; it helps get the body to where it needs to be.

During the Triple Dare, I lost three and three-quarter pounds. It doesn't sound like much, but those were stubborn pounds that I was trying to lose all last year.

Am I excited? Revved up? Ready to go? Feeling great? You bet I am! What really happened with me? I got risky in response to Carole's challenge and became a real daredevil. I dared to open up my heart to God in the previously closed area of exercise. And God answered that dare by helping me turn the page on old habits and begin again. He inspired me to use more music to put pep in my step and a new song in my heart. The memory verse CDs helped to put His Word deep inside me—walking and learning. A fresh start with exercise: God and I, walking together and working from the inside out. A different heartbeat that races toward the goal with Him, teaching me anew and creating more intimacy with Him. I am standing taller and straighter, carrying myself like the soldier I am in the army of the mighty King!

Do I dare step outside my comfort zone? Do I dare to be committed to God in all areas of my life? Do I dare to be different and honestly work from the inside out? As I put my hand, my heart, my soul, my body, my everything—yes, including my exercise—at His feet (making elbow prints on my bed), He and I work together for a holy, happy, healthy body that is ready and fit for service.

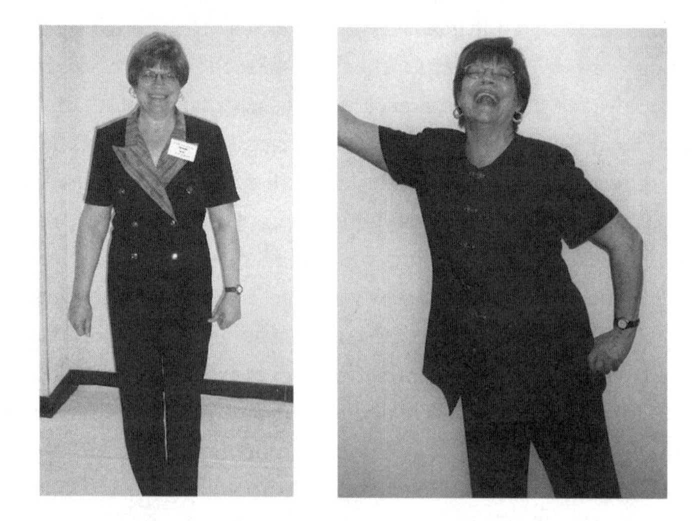

Dailiness is the answer: to open my heart to God and allow His miracle to work, to help me exercise because I want to do it for Him. Every day with Jesus! Dailiness journaling helps me look at yesterday for the lesson, use today for action and moving forward, and use tomorrow to pick up the challenges, knowing that God is the heartbeat of success to meet my goal.

Thank You, Jesus, for my dailiness miracle in exercise and the challenge of Triple Dare. I can do all things through You and with You. You are truly the only way to begin again—for commitments to be made, goals to be met and miracles to happen!

"Commit to the LORD whatever you do, and your plans will succeed" (Prov. 16:3).

ROB HEATH

HANAHAN, SOUTH CAROLINA

Father knows best, but sometimes, friends are pretty sharp, too!

I am rapidly approaching being a middle-aged pastor; I'm a father of four, who had a great father growing up. This helped me greatly when my earthly father introduced me to my heavenly Father. It was only natural that I would believe, trust and obey this heavenly Father—in many of the same ways that I had learned to trust my earthly father. I simply continued my conviction that father knows best—only with a new Father. Now in my late 40s, I've been sensing from my heavenly Father the need to address some health issues. I've been fairly active and I've made mostly good choices; but, frankly, I was a little short for my weight.

Fast forward to Round Top, Texas, site of First Place Fitness Week. Great environment; great friends (new and old); I'm there with my wife—life is good. Carole Lewis is looking for a few friends to make a fresh start and take the Triple Dare to really believe God in the area of personal health management. She tells her story; I listen and my flesh is interested—because I have a need—but my spirit is *not* willing. I have an excuse—

or two: The timing isn't good and I need to get some things in order before I start trying to address the habits and routine that have put about 19 pounds too many onto my 5′8″ preacher's frame. The night of decision comes. I am quiet and thinking, *I'll pass, this time, and no one will notice. Then later, perhaps in a week or two, I'll address my need.* My mind is wandering. Others in the room are responding, choosing; I've decided to wait until later.

Then, my thoughts are interrupted, and that winsome voice with the penetrating Texas drawl that can only belong to Carole Lewis says, "How about it, Rob, my man, are you in?" So, now I've got my own observation that I need to address some things; my heavenly Father is prompting me to address some things; and Carole Lewis is asking if I'm in. How would you respond? Well I gave it a thumbs up, of course. I had no idea just what God was up to; I was and am reminded that He not only knows *best,* but He also knows *more.*

By the end of Fitness Week, I had lost nearly 5 pounds. Afterward, I worked diligently, lived my commitments and made good progress right up to those last 4 or 5 pounds. Again, I focused and lived my commitments until the 19 pounds were history. Then, quite unexpectedly, two things hit me for a loop: I began an eight-week sabbatical, which

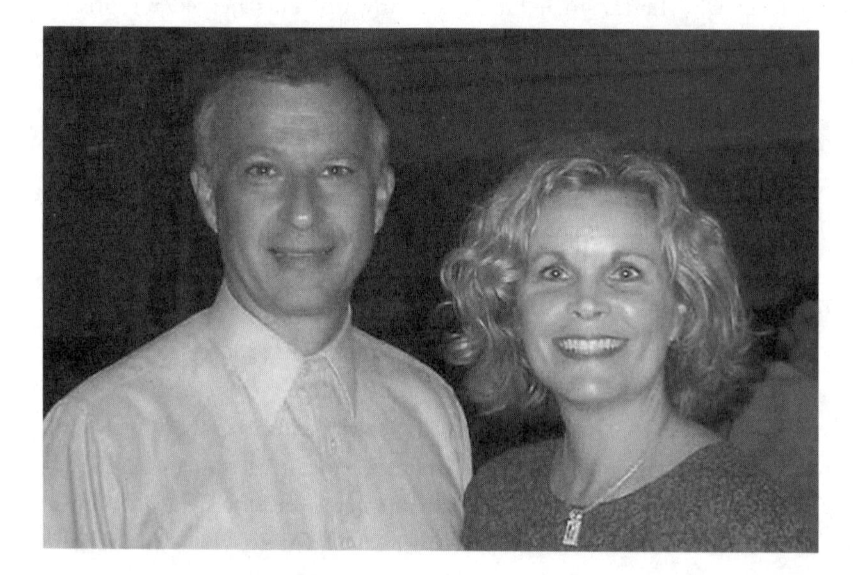

included a good deal of living out of a suitcase—a real challenge on the food-intake side of things; and I injured my knee—a badly strained medial collateral ligament. This radically altered what I could do for exercise. Predictably, I added back 4 or 5 pounds during this time, but I allowed and am continuing to allow my Father to teach me.

Now my knee has healed and I've restarted my jogging routine. I fully intend to get back to where I was—and I'll probably appreciate it more. And I'm so grateful that the 4 or 5 pounds I've gained were added to my new weight and not to the original. I would weigh more now than

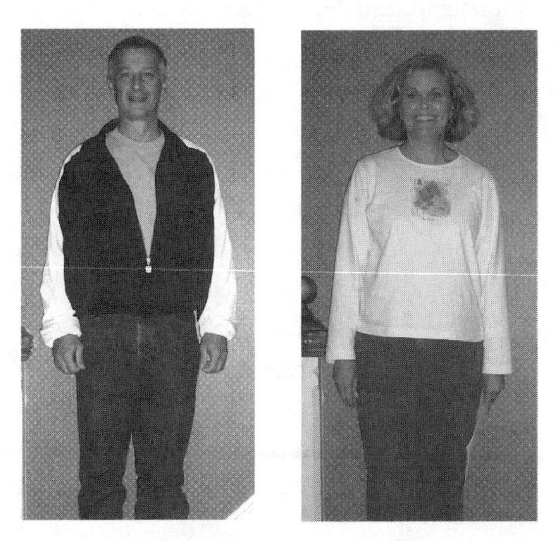

Rob's wife, Vicki, lost eight pounds on the Triple Dare.

I did before starting the Triple Dare had I not responded positively to my Father's timing and that penetrating Texas drawl asking "How about it, Rob, my man, are you in?"

Shelia Gross

Keithville, Louisiana

I've been in First Place for a little over 10 years. Spiritually, the Lord has changed my life completely; now I have a real relationship with Him, which I hadn't experienced before. But even though I've had this relationship with Christ, I haven't focused a lot on the physical part of my life. During the sessions, I'd faithfully follow the plan and lose weight; but when the sessions ended, I would gain back what I'd lost—only to have to begin again when the next session started. This was a vicious and unhealthy cycle.

It was at this time in my life that I went to the First Place conference in Hattiesburg, Mississippi. During the conference, God convicted me about my lack of commitment between sessions, but He added the final touch when Carole Lewis challenged us to take the Triple Dare.

I began this journey with no reservations in my heart. These 16 weeks have been challenging in many ways, but the Lord kept His promise that He would be with me during times of temptation and would provide a way out if I were willing to take it. I did great all during Thanksgiving and through Christmas. When I made all kinds of candies, pies and Christmas goodies during the days before Christmas, I would eat one piece occasionally (never more than one piece and not every day). And on Christmas Day, I didn't eat to the point of misery like I'd usually do (though I did eat a little more than I should have, and I ate a piece of pecan pie).

But the day after Christmas, I began to lose control. I'm not really sure what happened. I ate some desserts and several pieces of candy. For several days I would write in my journal that I needed to get back on track and that on that day I was going to begin again, but I didn't. Finally, on the morning of December 30, during my quiet time, God reminded me that I was doing this all wrong, that I couldn't get focused by myself but that with His help I could. I confessed my inability to Him.

At that point, I really did believe that I could get my focus back because of Him. Each time I was tempted, I would pray for strength and for the desire to stay focused and eat healthily. I'm thankful that God was faithful to help me. I regained my focus that day and have done well, losing 16¾ pounds and 14½ inches during the Triple Dare. I reached my overall goal.

I'm so thankful for the opportunity to go to the conference in Hattiesburg. It was through that conference and the Triple Dare that

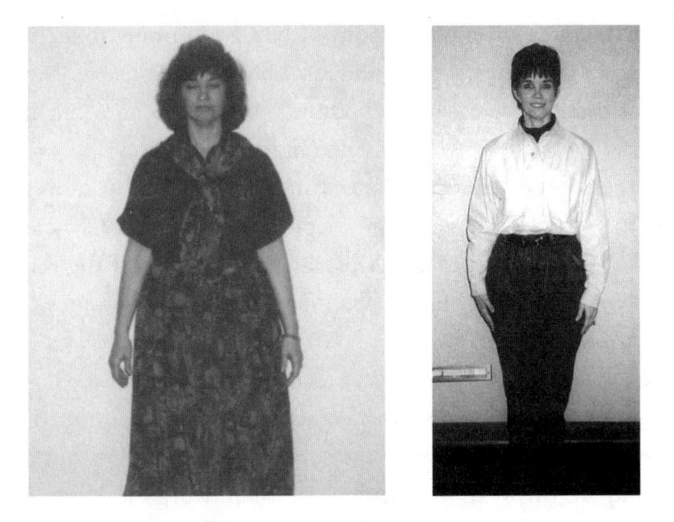

God helped me realize that I've only been playing at First Place, not really living it. Though it has taken me a little over 10 years, now I believe I can live it because of Christ and His faithfulness.

Tonia Price

Jackson, Mississippi

I would like to start my testimony by thanking God for introducing me to First Place and for what it has done in my life for the past two years.

I started First Place in January 2001. I lost 44 pounds and 20 inches within six months. My pictures and testimony were placed on Carol Moore's website at www.msfirstplace.com. I was able to keep my commitment with First Place until I found out we were moving.

We were finally settled May 2002, and I decided to get back on track—especially since I had gained 15 pounds. I struggled all during the summer and didn't do well at all. I looked for a First Place class where I now live but was unsuccessful in finding one. I needed something extra to help me.

I then heard about the conference that was going to be held in September 2002, in Hattiesburg, Mississippi. I knew that I had to get the weight back off, especially since people there probably would have seen my pictures and read my testimony—I had an example to set with my weight loss. I got back on track and lost about 6 pounds before the conference. I didn't lose all the 15 pounds, but the 6 sure did help my appearance, because I am tall and can hide the weight well.

While at the conference, Miss Carole challenged those of us who are not on maintenance to take the Triple Dare. Though I had been on maintenance, I decided to take this challenge to get off the rest of the weight I had gained. I knew I needed this to help me, since I hadn't found a class yet.

The Triple Dare definitely was a challenge for me, but the Lord never gave up on me. I kept up with the daily journal and continued to pray for guidance. I decided not to worry about my weight loss but to focus on shaping up this year. My exercise had mainly been walking, but now I have added jogging and TaeBo, and I want to start doing some floor exercises.

The Triple Dare was what I needed to get me back on track. I lost five pounds, which got me back to my maintenance goal, but I did not lose any inches. However, I hope to lose inches as I continue to shape up and to make First Place a lifetime commitment. The Lord has been so good to me to introduce me to First Place. First Place has been my way of making a lifetime commitment to God and to myself.

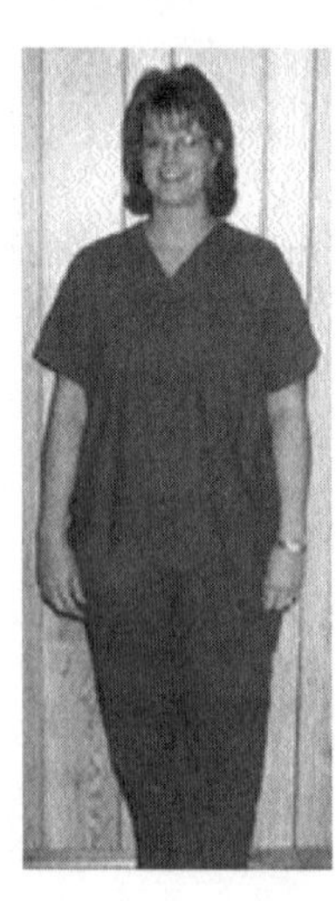

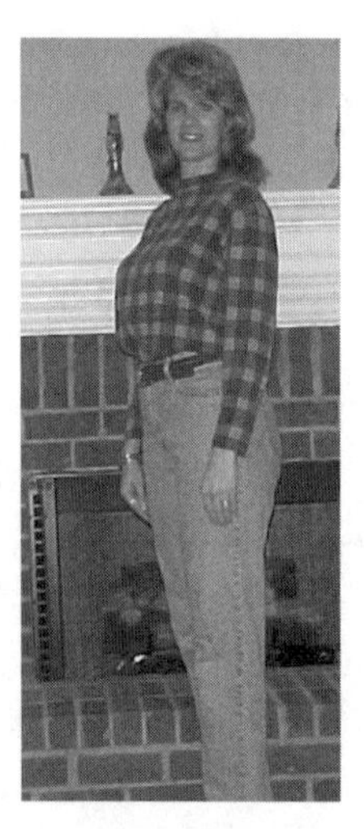

I would like to add one other struggle that I've been dealing with recently. I've been in desperate need of a part-time job, and I had the chance of getting one with a local weight-loss group that does not acknowledge what God can do in our weight-loss battle. Though it was a difficult decision to make, I decided not to take the job, because God deserves all the credit for what He can and will do in our lives. He has a job out there waiting for me—I'll just wait.

NOTES

Chapter 1

1. Ron Kurtus, "Winston Churchill's 'Never Give Up' Speech," *School for Champions,* May 20, 2001. http://www.school-for-champions.com/speeches/churchill_never giveup.htm (accessed February 10, 2003).

Chapter 3

1. Zig Ziglar, *See You at the Top* (New York: Pelican Publishing Company, 1975), p. 231.

Chapter 5

1. Oswald Chambers, *My Utmost for His Highest: An Updated Edition in Today's Language,* ed. James Reimann (Grand Rapids, MI: Discovery House Publishers, 1992), reading for November 5.
2. Charlie Plum, interview by Dr. James Dobson, *Focus on the Family*, KSBJ FM, Houston, TX, November 7, 2002.

Chapter 6

1. "A Quiz," *Laugh and Lift,* November 5, 2002. http://www.laughandlift.com/lift347.html (accessed February 17, 2003).

Chapter 7

1. Joseph M. Stowell, *Strength for the Journey* (Chicago, IL: Moody Press, 2002), p. 323.

Chapter 11

1. Stowell, *Strength for the Journey,* p. 342.

Chapter 13

1. Ziglar, *See You at the Top,* p. 238.